KV-203-566

BRAIN INJURY

– TAPPING THE POTENTIAL WITHIN –

Treatment and Progress through Stimulation,
Movement and Love

Ian Hunter

Collaborating Editor:
Barbara Muhvich

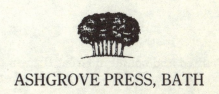

ASHGROVE PRESS, BATH

First published in Great Britain by
ASHGROVE PRESS LIMITED
19 Circus Place, Bath, Avon BA1 2PW

© Ian Hunter, 1986, 1987

Originally published in Australia by
Hill of Content Publishing Company Pty Ltd

This edition published 1987

British Library Cataloguing in Publication Data

Hunter, Ian
  Brain injury: tapping the potential within.
  1. Mentally handicapped children—Care and
  treatment
  I. Title   II. Muhvich, Barbara
  362.3′088054   HV891

  ISBN 0-906798-78-7
  ISBN 0-906798-75-2 Pbk

Printed and bound in Great Britain by
Biddles Ltd, Guildford and King's Lynn

BRAIN INJURY –
TAPPING THE POTENTIAL WITHIN

The following pages are particularly addressed to those whose child, friend or patient is described as being:

cerebral palsied;
spastic;
athetoid;
mentally retarded;
autistic;
developmentally delayed;
intellectually handicapped;
slow learning;
learning disabled;
dyslexic;
hyperactive;
epileptic.

CONTENTS

FOREWORD

For several decades, the brain injured child has been an enigma to both the medical profession and to parents. There has been little real understanding of the problem, and the results of treatments used for the most part have been disappointing.

Instead of saying that past failures only go to prove that little can be done to help the tragic victims of brain injury, we have to look again at how this problem can best be treated. This is precisely what Ian Hunter has done in writing this book. *Brain Injury – Tapping the Potential Within* encompasses the logic, importance and scientific aspects of a sound neurophysiological approach to the treament of the brain injured child.

We have spent our professional lives teaching, amongst other things, one simple fact to doctors, therapists and parents from all around the world – that brain injury lies within the brain. If the treatment of this often devastating problem is to be successful, all efforts need to be directed to the brain rather than to the peripheral symptoms. With fifty-five years of combined experience of using these principles, we have been most encouraged by the results of our work with brain injured children.

Ian Hunter, our student and colleague for eleven years, has clearly outlined the concepts, philosophies and methodology necessary for sound neurophysiological treatment. He backs up this approach with scientific evidence, logic and experience.

This is an important book for professionals working in the field of brain injury. More importantly, it is a book for parents who are looking for answers. For the most part, these parents have been led to believe that it is extremely difficult, if not impossible, to significantly change the function of an injured brain. However, as this book so clearly demonstrates, we now know that brain growth and development are not static – but comprise a dynamic process that can be affected in both negative and, more importantly, positive ways. In simple and understandable language, Ian Hunter shows how it is possible to enhance the function of the brain, even after severe brain injury.

Throughout the years, we have seen innumerable parents who have not been satisfied with the treatment made available to their children, or with the progress – or lack of progress – that these treatments have achieved. These parents are seeking more knowledge, different approaches and improved results. Like Ian Hunter, we have devoted our lives to this endeavour. Now, the answers to many of their questions, along with an explanation of a feasible and reasonable alternative form of treatment, can be found in this book.

We wish to congratulate our former student, not only for his continued determination and excellent work with brain injured children in Australia, but also for this outstanding book. We hope and pray that many children will be able to take advantage of this exciting new approach because of this book.

Art Sandler,
Sandra Brown,
Sandler Brown Consultants,
Willow Grove, Pennsylvania, U.S.A.

ACKNOWLEDGEMENTS

To the parents who so generously contributed their stories, I give my sincere thanks.

I also wish to express particular gratitude to my wife, Sharron, to my collaborating editor, Barbara Muhvich, and to Gary Satherley, Dr Ted Freeman, Dr Jane Lees-Millais and Dr Barry Ryan.

Special acknowledgement is made to Dr Marshall Mandell for contributing the chapter on the relationship between brain injury and allergies.

To Art Sandler and Sandra Brown of Sandler-Brown Rehabilitation Consultants, Philadelphia, world leaders in the type of treatment described in this book, thank you for writing the foreword and for your guidance over the years.

Ian Hunter

To the children and their parents

This book is dedicated in the hope that each
parent can find the strength and the energy
needed to help their brain injured child reach
his or her potential, whatever that potential may be.

Happy are those who dream dreams,
and are ready to pay the price to
make them come true
                    L. J. Cardinal Suenens

Two Eyes, Two Hands, Two Feet . . .

THE unspoken fear of most expecting parents is that there might be something wrong with their baby, that it won't fit into society's concept of what is 'normal'. So strong is this emotion that, when asked whether they would prefer a boy or girl, most parents-to-be respond by saying they don't really care – all they want is a healthy, normal baby.

Immediately after the child is born, most parents are anxious to be alone with their baby. They like to make sure for themselves that everything is all right. At this time, they usually conduct a physical inventory: 'Two eyes, two hands, two feet . . .'

Their concern does not end at the baby's birth. Indeed, it has only just begun! Every high fever, every childhood illness, every serious fall or accident will be accompanied by the inevitable question: 'Will our child be all right?'

Most parents will never have to live through the anguish and despair of finding out that their child is not normal. They will not experience the unavoidable feelings of guilt, nor the need to try and blame somebody or something. They will never truly understand the feeling of hopelessness that hangs over the family of the child which is not normal. Yet, for many, this scenario will be their nightmare reality. The statistics show that it happens to a greater number of people than most would suspect. In Britain, for example, it is estimated that one baby in every 400 will be born with brain injury resulting in cerebral palsy.[1] One child in every 660 will suffer from Down's Syndrome.[2] One child in 2,500 will be autistic.[3]

In 1987 Mencap estimated that one in 100 children in the UK were being born with a mental handicap, that is twenty per day, and that there were 500,000 people of all ages in the country suffering from mental handicap,[4] one third of whom might be classified as severely handicapped.[4]

In the United States of America, the United Cerebral Palsy Association has estimated that there are 500,000 to 700,000 people suffering from one or more symptoms of cerebral palsy. In addition, 7,000 to 9,000 children are born with cerebral palsy each year, and another 1,200 to 1,500 pre-school children become cerebral palsied annually as a result of brain injury from accidents and infections.[5]

The incidence of brain injury resulting from some kind of trauma or illness that occurs at any stage after birth is also much higher than expected. The Australian Brain Foundation reports that every year, more than 40,000 Australians of all ages go to hospital with some kind of head injury – although the vast majority of these injuries cause no serious long-term problems.[6] In the United States, the National Head Injury Foundation has estimated that each year, following head injury, between 50,000 to 90,000 people are left with intellectual and behavioural deficits of such a degree as to preclude their return to normal life. Two thirds of these people are below the age of 30.[7] Other genetic, developmental, or unspecified defects and injuries of the brain will account for thousands and thousands of children around the world each year. The problem is immense.

The financial side of brain injury also has to be considered. Dr Noel Dan, Chairman of the Trauma Sub-committee of the Neurosurgical Society of Australasia[8], estimated that neurotrauma (trauma to the brain, spinal cord and peripheral nerves) cost the state of New South Wales almost $1 billion in 1977, and Australia $3 billion. If it were possible to calculate the ongoing treatment and welfare costs of children born with brain injury, and if this figure was added to the costs of those brain injured through trauma, the final total would be astronomical.

Of course, nobody can even begin to calculate the hidden cost of brain injury – the human suffering of not only those directly affected, but also that of their families and friends. This aspect alone makes brain injury a problem of major proportions.

Despite its obvious extent, brain injury is an issue that most of us have shied away from. We have thought: 'It's not my problem, and since I am not affected by it, I'd rather not become involved. Besides, it's too depressing to even think about.' Perhaps we have thought that by looking the other way, brain injured people will somehow disappear. Even better, if we put them into institutions, they can be conveniently forgotten.

In primitive cultures, some brain injured children die due to the absence of appropriate medical care. Others are sometimes left to die as an act of mercy. In these harsh environments, survival of the fittest is a rule of life – there is no alternative. Likewise, many animals will starve their young if they sense that something is wrong.

In some ways, our civilized culture has not done much better. The policy of keeping some brain injured children in institutions has done little to improve their condition, since in these establishments the patient is just given basic care rather than intensive treatment. It is not only the patients who have been adversely affected by such an approach, for many families have suffered great heartache in having to give up children that they love. Even today, some parents of brain injured children are presented with no option to putting their child away into an institution.

It is difficult enough for parents to just come to terms with the fact that their child is brain injured, let alone to be told that the best thing to do is to hand over the child to the authorities so that they can care for him for the rest of his life.

With the news that their child is brain injured, most parents first go through a grieving stage, dealing with issues such as accepting that their child has a problem which no amount of wishful thinking will eradicate. They also must come to terms with feelings of guilt, and the impression that life has dealt them, and their child, an unfair blow. The length of this grieving period varies. Some parents quickly come to terms with their child's problems, others may take several years. A few never seem to reach this point, a tragedy for all concerned.

After acceptance of the child's problem, parents naturally want to find out how they can improve the situation. It seems logical to them that once the problem has been detected, attempts should be made to try and rectify it.

Herein lies the biggest problem of all – finding out what can best be done to help their child. For many parents, this is where the heartache really begins, because, even though their child may have been diagnosed as being brain injured, it doesn't necessarily mean a solution will be given. In fact, many are told that there is little or nothing that can be done, especially if their child is severely brain injured. Children as young as six months have been virtually written off as being hopeless, and their parents have been told that there is little point in doing any kind of therapy – at six months!

Time and time again, parents are told that there are no answers, that the best thing they can do is take their child home and love him the way he is. They are also warned not to expect too much improvement. Parents can learn to accept that their child is brain injured, but many *cannot* accept that nothing can be done.

It is this implied permanence which makes the prospect of having a brain injured child such a daunting one. Brain injury seems to be unlike many of the other things that can go wrong with children. For instance, if a child breaks a leg, as unpleasant and inconvenient as it may be, it is not usually an injury of lasting consequences. In most cases, the break will heal properly with appropriate medical care.

Such is not the case with brain injury – or so the world thinks. No one really imagines that a spastic child can develop near-normal movement ability, or that a mentally retarded child can significantly improve his intellectual capacity.

Most of us have the preconceived notion that the condition of brain injury is permanent, with little or no possibility for improvement. This is what makes a pregnant woman worry when she wonders what her baby will be like; this is what makes the mother of a normal child panic when her child has a severe virus, or gets hit on the head; and this is what concerns a doctor when a brain injured child comes into his office for the first time, for he knows that medicine does not have many answers for these children.

Yet, we believe that there *are* some answers; not for every child perhaps, but certainly for a great many.

Parents of brain injured children treated by the Australian Centre for Brain Injured Children recently responded to a survey aimed at assessing the benefits of a therapy program based on the concepts presented in this book. Of the 154 respondents, eighty-three said that the treatment was 'very beneficial'. A further forty-three rated it as having been 'moderately beneficial'. Therefore, in the eyes of the parents, 82 per cent of the patients made moderate to very beneficial progress (see Appendix One).

We feel that these are excellent results, especially when it is realized that many of the children treated had already undergone 'conventional' treatment without success. As well, in some cases, the parents were advised that their child's problems were so severe that no amount of therapy would make any difference. It certainly did make a difference – to a significant degree in 82 per cent of the children.

In these pages, we trust that you will find hope for the future of your brain injured child, friend, relative, or patient.

Section I
The Situation Today

CHAPTER ONE

It Couldn't Happen to Us

NOTHING can match the heartache, nor the mental anguish, that parents live through when they come to realize that their precious baby or child is not quite normal. A mental or physical problem may have been detected; but what is its cause? How bad is it? What will be its ultimate effects? How can it be treated?

Then there is the frustration and the overwhelming feeling of hopelessness that comes from unsuccessfully seeking answers to these questions. There is the despair of being told there is no hope, that nothing can be done to help the child. And there is sorrow, guilt, fear, jealousy, hate, love – all powerful emotions, all churning within a heart that feels as if it is being torn apart.

But try as one might, someone who is not actually a parent of a brain injured child cannot possibly imagine what it is really like. So that we can better understand their anguish and despair, and just what they have to cope with, we have asked several parents of brain injured children to describe their early experiences. Their stories follow, and in the final chapter of this book, the same parents will relate, in much happier terms, how their children have improved, despite the gloomy pictures that were painted for each of them.

Chantal Coates

Chantal Coates is now five years old, and lives in Cairns, Queensland. Her parents are Kerrie and Denis. Kerrie writes:

The day finally arrives when we hear the words we have been dreading for the last sad six months. Six months of hurt, bewilderment, constant anger, depression, and, most of all, the never-ending questions raging in our minds, asking what happened to cause the hurt to our little baby.

The doctor is saying: 'I'm sorry Mr and Mrs Coates, but your daughter is severely retarded. She is cortically blind, and it is most unlikely that she will ever develop a mentality beyond that of a one year old'.

These words are like a life sentence to us. No judge or jury could have delivered a worse punishment. Our happy lives changed so dramatically and destructively, all in a mere fifteen seconds.

Just six months ago, we were a contented young family of four, eagerly awaiting our new arrival. Chantal was a seemingly normal baby for the first six days of her life. Let me remember the morning we brought our wonderful little girl home from the hospital . . .

Although she was our third child, it felt no different to when we brought our first one home. How proud we were! How our love surged as we continually ran to see our little princess laying in her emerald green bassinet. That night I went to bed secure and content in the thought of how complete my little world felt.

Any new mother feels tired at the six a.m. feed, and I don't claim to be any different. But, my tiredness gave way to panic and fear as I watched in horror – a very strange and alien movement occurred all over my baby's tiny body whilst I cradled her in my arms.

She was gasping, her mouth opening and closing – like a fish out of water. Her whole body was in a horrible rhythm, writhing to some ghastly tune that only she could hear.

A nurse had been staying at our home looking after our other children while I was in hospital having Chantal. She came into the bedroom in response to my screams, and was just in time to see the last of the baby's grotesque movements. She tried to reassure me, saying that it was probably just a normal reflex that was nothing to worry about.

But the horror of what I had witnessed remained firmly planted in my mind. It surfaced again in a heartbreaking flood at the ten a.m. feed, when, once again I was the unwilling witness to my baby's terrifying squirming.

All I remember of the following nightmare drive to the hospital, holding my sleeping angel in my arms, was a feeling of crushing weakness and utter despair. I was afraid, I pleaded silently and desperately: 'Please God, just let my baby live. I don't care what happens to me, all I want is for my baby to survive'.

My husband, Denis, rushed to my side at the hospital. The whole day spent there was one of sheer helplessness and utter despair. Chantal underwent tests that left her hoarse from screaming.

It took several abortive attempts to do a proper lumbar puncture, and to do this, they had to roll my small, sick, six-day-old baby into a ball. We watched her angry little body twist and turn as she cried, but no sound came from her. It was a heart-breaking sight, more than we could bear. We cried with her.

Chantal stayed in hospital for three weeks as intensive tests were carried out, and we kept a constant vigil by her bedside, only returning home to sleep. At this stage, I couldn't bear to see her bassinet and clothing, so I put them away. It was almost as if she didn't exist any more.

At the end of the tests, the doctors told us that the horrible movements that I had seen Chantal make were, in fact, a type of seizure or epilepsy. At this point they weren't sure if they were going to continue, or if they would affect her development.

What then followed can be best described as 'the waiting game'. The doctors didn't actually use these words, but that is how we interpreted their attitude. The next three to four months involved an agony of waiting for normal development to occur, while at the same time desperately hoping that this would in fact happen.

We kept asking: 'Why can't we *do* something to help her?' But the answer always was: 'The only thing you can do is *wait*'.

I had gone into shock after Chantal's first seizure, and I walked around like a zombie. All my reflexes slowed down, I had a thick feeling in my tongue, and I was constantly sleepy. It was like being heavily sedated. I thank God that I was affected like this, for I don't think that I could have coped any other way.

Denis was a tower of strength, and he bore his hurt and bewilderment with gentle courage. These are qualities I have always loved in him and always will.

With a cloud of gloom still hanging over us, it was so difficult to return to normal life. Going to playgroup with my other children was a harsh experience. I felt jealousy towards other babies who had been born around the same time as Chantal. It cut me like a knife when all the mothers gathered around admiring the 'normal' babies, while I stood alone with my physically beautiful, but brain injured, daughter.

I suppose they didn't want to upset me by talking about her and the problems she had, and yet, this is what I needed most of all. Just a few sympathetic ears so I could release all that pent-up hurt and frustration. Oh, how I needed to talk at that time!

Instead, I retreated into my shell with all my negative thoughts. 'What will her future be? How will we bear it when she is sixteen or seventeen years old, so beautiful in face and body, but with nothing at all in her mind?'

Again and again, I remembered the doctor's damning sentence: 'I am sorry Mr and Mrs Coates, but Chantal is severely retarded . . . cortically blind . . . she'll never develop a mentality beyond that of a one year old'.

How very wrong this proved to be.

Ryan Cuthill

Ryan is five years old, and lives in Sydney. His parents are Jan and Ray. Jan writes:

Ryan's arrival was of particular joy to Ray and I, as although I had to have fertility treatment before the birth of the other two children, we had conceived Ryan spontaneously. As well, we had lost our third baby only four hours after birth.

On the day that he arrived, I had a surprise visit from the hospital paediatrician. I was certainly not expecting the news that followed, for he told me that I had a very sick little baby. He was convulsing, and they had to give him medication to stop this. He also was being given oxygen as he was having breathing difficulties. Unless Ryan settled down soon, the paediatrician was going to have to consult with specialists at the major children's hospital.

I went into deep shock. I had lost one baby, and didn't think I could cope with losing another one. The next few days were absolute hell. I felt worse than normal after the caesarean because of the shock. My muscles became weak and jelly-like and they didn't seem to want to coordinate. Ray was a great comfort to me in those first few days, and all through our battle with Ryan. I suppose that we were a comfort to each other.

Eventually, after six long days, the paediatrician informed us that Ryan was being sent to the Children's Hospital, because he could not do without the medication and he still needed oxygen. This was the last straw. I broke down and howled. Everything that had been building up inside since Ryan was born just came flooding out.

Once Ryan was taken to the other hospital, I was allowed to go home. Ray and I talked about what had happened and what lay ahead. We wondered why this had happened to us, why other people seem to go through life without all the problems that we had been confronted with. But we did not dwell in self-pity – instead, we decided to get on with doing something about it. We made a pact there and then: 'We are not going to let this beat us'.

It was not until Ryan was thirteen days old that I was able to actually hold him, but even then, we were separated from each other by the walls of the humidicrib in which he had to stay. With tubes and wires attached to his body and an oxygen mask under his nose, I had my first cuddle. I felt like a mother at last as the love flowed through me to this helpless little bundle. Those wretched holes in the humidicrib through which we were able to touch and feel were vile.

For five weeks I went to the hospital daily with my expressed milk, as he was too weak to try on the breast. We grew to love this little mite. Our other children came along too and, along with Dad, they had their turn to cuddle him. We noticed that Ryan responded to the children and to our voices, and this naturally thrilled us.

The worst thing during this time was not knowing what was wrong with him. All the tests showed nothing, and the doctors were bamboozled. They discovered a small hole in his heart, but they weren't sure if this was what was causing his breathing problems.

One day, I was so depressed and miserable, and as I left the hospital, I could feel tears running down my face. As I drove out of the car park, there before me was the massive brick wall of the Weston's biscuit factory. I looked at it and thought: 'I would like to drive this car into that wall and end it all – this heartache, this hell I am going through'.

I don't know how I stopped myself. I guess it was the thought of Ray and the other children. Somehow, I managed to drive past that wall instead of into it.

Finally, I was able to try breast feeding. But what a let down after waiting for so long, for Ryan had enormous problems trying to suck properly. By the time we tried all the different techniques of getting his mouth open and then getting the nipple in, the sucking that took place wasn't strong enough. He would then have to be tube fed, as he wasn't taking enough of my milk. Mothers usually have happy memories of breast feeding, but mine are the exact opposite.

After many frustrating days, we succeeded in giving him my expressed milk in a bottle, and we were eventually able to remove the tube. At last, now the tube was removed, the doctors said that we could take Ryan home, as he would be better off with the stimulation of a normal house and his family.

The day I was to pick him up, I was so nervous that I didn't know what I was doing. I didn't know how I was going to cope, but I was determined to make him better.

Everything was alright for the first couple of weeks, as he continued to feed well on his bottles of expressed milk. However, it didn't last long, as for some reason his sucking ability went backwards. It now took two hours to feed him, and I had to encourage his swallowing by poking his cheeks and tickling him under the chin, as well as dabbing his face with a wet washer to keep him awake. Luckily, I met a social worker by chance at the hospital, and she recommended a squeeze bottle. It worked! The social worker was surprised that no one had given me one before, but this was typical of the way I was left to my own devices to find solutions to all these problems I had to deal with.

At five months of age, I could see that Ryan wasn't developing normally. He was as floppy as a rag doll – he couldn't even hold his head up. I felt that the sooner I did something to help him the better, so I talked to the paediatrician.

He agreed with me, but wanted to do more tests to see if his problem could be diagnosed.

More tests! The uncertainty of it all was unnerving. No one knew how long he would live, or whether his problems would get better or worse. They didn't even know what exactly was wrong with him.

All I wanted was to start doing something to help him. This time I asked the paediatrician about therapy, and he referred me to a physiotherapist. This was the beginning of our long, slow battle to help Ryan become as normal as possible.

At this stage, I knew nothing about his severe scoliosis – a curvature of the spine. The physiotherapist noticed it and suggested that I see an orthopaedic specialist about it. I had noticed that Ryan was asymmetrical, but I thought that this was due to the chest deformities I knew he had. It was such a shock to find out that there was yet another thing wrong with Ryan. I started to feel unsure about the doctors.

Were they holding things back from me? What else would we find wrong that we didn't know about?

When I saw a doctor, I now started asking as many questions as possible, and if I felt the question was being evaded, or not given a satisfactory answer, I asked it in a different way. I needed to have the whole story.

By this time, I was getting extremely frustrated and desperate as Ryan just wasn't making any improvement at all. What a trying time. I didn't think we were going to get anywhere – but our faith in God helped us through. I believe that God helps those who help themselves, and this is why I did not sit and wait for help to come. Instead, I went after it and was willing to try anything that might help my child – even when conventional medicine sneered at my decision to try an unorthodox method of treatment.

Terese Gage

Terese is also five years old, and she lives in Sydney. Her parents are Kris and Rob. Kris writes:

When Terese was born, we were so overjoyed at having a girl, since our first child was a boy. They put her down on my tummy, and we thought she was beautiful – although we both made comments at the time that she was funny looking in some way. I put this down to never having seen a baby in its first moments after birth. I remember Rob saying: 'You are beautiful, but you'll never win a beauty contest!'

We were oblivious to it then, but later we recalled that the nurses and doctors weren't excited about the birth. Almost immediately, the intern asked us which paediatrician we would like. Even then we weren't worried, as we thought that this was just normal practice.

While I was cleaned up, my husband went off to break the good news to family and friends. I was put in another room for a while and lay there crying with happiness. I remember thinking: 'I can't wait for my mother to hold my little one', as we had always been close and I knew she would be thrilled that we'd had a girl.

Not long after, as I lay there contentedly thinking of the joys that lay ahead with our little girl, the replacement doctor for my own gynaecologist came to see me. What he had to say completely devastated me – he said that things weren't at all well and that there was a lot of cause for concern. It seemed that our baby had rather an odd shaped head.

I was absolutely shattered. I broke down and just wanted to see my husband. Words could never explain the extent of the empty, horrifying feeling I was experiencing. The bottom just fell out of my world.

As they were ringing my husband, a nursing sister came and tried to comfort me. She was the first one to mention the word 'retarded', and it really started to hit home just what it all meant. After my husband arrived, we had to wait almost ten hours to see the paediatrician. Every minute seemed like an hour, and we both felt sick, empty and alone as we waited and waited.

The doctor finally arrived, and he told us that our precious baby was 'microcephalic'. He explained that this meant that her head was small, probably because of something that had happened to the brain. It was not very reassuring to hear that he was currently dealing with another microcephalic patient, a five-year-old who had just been put into an institution.

It was sheer hell and torture hearing all the things that could go wrong with our ltitle girl. I remember lying in bed that night picturing a little figure lying on the floor, unable to do anything. I had requested to be moved into a room by myself, as I couldn't stand being with the other mothers and seeing them so happy.

Looking back, I don't know if that was such a good thing, as I had so much time to myself. Time to torture myself with questions like: 'Why me? Why us? What did I do wrong? How could it have happened?' I kept asking: 'What will she be like? What will she do?' But nobody could give me any answers. I would just have to wait and see.

I just wanted it to be a nightmare. I wanted to wake up and find it wasn't really happening. Then, the sick, empty feeling inside came back with a vengeance as I realized it wasn't a dream.

I finally took my baby home on the sixth day after birth. It certainly was a different feeling to that when I brought my first baby home. I found the nights the worst, as I would lay awake thinking. It was so hard not knowing what she was going to be like, or what exactly was wrong, or even if she could be helped in any way. I remember feeling very bitter when I went shopping and saw all the normal children, especially the pretty little girls.

And yet, right from when we brought Terese home, she was alert and her eyes were bright. We took her for check-ups, but the news was always so gloomy: 'There is something wrong, but we don't know how bad she will be. We will just have to wait and see'. As the weeks went by we recovered a little, but the hardest thing to accept was that nothing could be done.

When Terese was nearly three months old, my aunt came to visit. She brought with her our first ray of hope. She told us that she was involved in helping a brain injured child who was undergoing a home therapy program, and she thought that this type of treatment might help Terese.

We were *so* excited, and we just couldn't believe it. This was like a dream come true – there *was* something that may help our little girl.

We found out more about this program, and even went to see some of the children who were doing it. We saw that there was some hope. At last, we were able to look forward to the future. So too were our families.

We haven't looked back since.

CHAPTER TWO

What's Wrong with Our Child?

IN THE first weeks of life, a baby is thoroughly scrutinized by his parents. They probably give him the best neurological assessment available. They are looking for any untoward sign which may indicate that something might be wrong, and they will ask themselves hundreds of questions as they observe their child's behaviour and development. Is he sucking properly? Are his hearing and eyesight normal? Should I call the doctor about that lump on his head?

This anxiety is simply part of being a parent. It is not that parents really want to find something wrong, but they know that if something is slightly amiss and is not detected, there could be drastic consequences. With subsequent children, this worry usually diminishes, although parents never really become complacent.

It seems logical to assume that, since parents act as natural 'early screening devices', they will usually be the first to detect the symptoms of brain injury. We have found this to be true.

As part of the parent survey mentioned in the Introduction, parents of children who were brain injured from birth, i.e. those whose brain injury did not occur as a result of an accident after birth, were asked the following questions: 'Who first detected the child's problem? When was this first noticed?' The answers to the questions are listed in Tables 1 and 2.

As can be seen, in over two-thirds of the children, the problem was first detected by the parents. When the parents were the first ones to notice that something was wrong, in nearly half of the cases this occurred before the child was six months old. By the time the child was twelve months old, 78 per cent of the parents suspected that the child was not developing normally.

What alerted these parents to suspect that their child had a problem? None were experts in child development, and many were first

Table 1: Who detected the problem?

	Detected by parent	By professional	By other family	Total
Number	69	25	6	100
%	69	25	6	

time parents. Most significantly, subsequent tests proved that their initial fears were correct. So, how did they know?

According to these parents, one of the most common signs first observed was that the baby wasn't sucking properly. From the first feed, the suck didn't feel as strong as they had expected, and each feed took a long time. Sucking is a very basic, primitive reflex, obviously vital for survival, and its development occurs while the baby is still in the womb. A twenty-week-old fetus, when touched around the lip area, responds by protruding the lips. By thirty-three weeks, the same light touching in the lip area causes the tongue to move out and along the lower lip. Since the sucking reflex develops before birth, a newborn should have a strong suck that begins immediately he is placed on the breast.

The absence or limited ability of such a vital reflex is a possible indicator that something may be wrong. This does not mean that every mother of a newborn who is not sucking properly should immediately suspect brain injury, as there are many children who do not suck very well at birth and yet develop normally. Like most indicators of brain injury, there is not a 100 per cent correlation. But poor sucking should be recognized as a possible early warning sign, especially if the baby's sucking ability does not improve with time. If the mother is breastfeeding, she may think that her baby's feeding problems are related to her milk supply, and this is sometimes the case. But, it is often directly related to the baby's poor sucking ability.

Another early sign of brain injury that has been noticed by parents is a poor sleep pattern. This type of problem can vary greatly, with the most obvious abnormality being a child who sleeps very poorly. In the first weeks of life, most babies sleep for most of the day and night. If the baby just has continual little cat naps, or is very difficult to get to sleep, this may indicate that the child has a problem. However, there are many factors which could cause a baby to sleep poorly, so parents should not see this as a definite sign of brain

Table 2: When did parents first detect the problem?

	Within six months	6-12 months	After 12 months	Total
Number	29	25	15	69
%	42	36	22	

injury. Rather, as with poor sucking, it should be recognized as another possible early indicator of brain injury.

Another problem related to sleep may not even be thought of as a sign that something may be wrong. You would not think that any fault could be found in an infant who sleeps so well that he usually has to be woken for feeds, and who, if left alone, would probably sleep almost all day and night. However, babies and infants should wake with hunger, and they are meant to stay awake for part of each day so that they can begin to explore the world around them. There is such a thing as a baby being 'too good' – so any baby who is content to sleep all of the time should be carefully looked at.

An abnormality in crying is another possible warning sign that warrants investigation. All babies should cry, some louder than others, and some more often. Unfortunately for their parents, the babies who cry the most are usually also the ones that cry the loudest. They have had lots of practice, and have found it to be a wonderfully effective way of attracting attention. Some children are naturally more frequent criers, while others are quite content and don't have the need to cry very often. Crying is a natural response to situations such as hunger, fear and discomfort, and should be used by the baby to express these needs or emotions. Apart from a child who cries almost continuously, other deviations from normal may include any unusual sounding cry, or a child who cries very little or not at all.

Within the first couple of months, most parents feel that they are communicating with their baby. But sometimes, parents feel that their baby doesn't seem as aware or as responsive as they would have expected, or that the bonding emotion isn't as strong as it has been with their other children. Something just doesn't seem right – it is nothing specific, but rather a deep-down feeling that they are not getting through to their baby.

Another comment that parents have made is that when they are holding or changing their baby, his body feels a little funny. His arms and legs may be a little stiff, or too loose. All children have different muscle and bone structures, but a baby should have a good range of movement in all his joints, without any apparent tightness or floppiness.

To reassure parents whose babies may have one of the problems mentioned, it is important to note that most parents who correctly detected early warning signs of brain injury in their children found that these signs usually occurred in combination. For instance, the child who sucked poorly cried a lot, and was a poor sleeper; or another who cried very little also slept most of the day, often had to be woken for feeds, and his body felt very floppy.

One of these signs in isolation is less likely to be an indicator of brain injury than several occurring together. Even so, each should be carefully investigated, just to be on the safe side. If several of these signs are present, this does not automatically mean the child is brain injured, though it would certainly warrant extensive testing.

* * *

Most of the parents who detect something wrong with their child within the first twelve months say that they are usually confronted with a frustrating problem after their discovery – that of finding someone who will listen to them. Often, their fears are dismissed as being those of over-anxious parents. From their doctors, they often get a standard response – they are told that all children develop at different rates, that their child is just a slow developer, that they are really too close to have an objective view. 'There is nothing to worry about, so why don't you come back in a couple of months?' is not uncommon advice.

Parents may visit many different doctors and specialists without satisfaction. Some may be lucky to find a doctor who recognizes the parents' role in early detection, and who takes careful notice of what they say. Unfortunately, this happens in only a minority of cases. More often, the parents' frustration gradually increases after each disappointing visit to a doctor. They ask each other in desperation: 'Why won't somebody listen to us? We know there is something wrong with our baby, and we want to know exactly what it is, so we can do everything possible to help him'.

But in most cases, no one hears. If only someone would. Then parents would be able to get their child properly examined and find out whether their fears are unfounded, or, in fact, there is something wrong.

Some medical practitioners adopt a protective attitude towards parents. For example, if the child is not performing as well as he should, as long as he is not too far behind his peers, it may seem best not to say anything to the parents as it could cause them unnecessary worry. What if the child is simply a slow developer who will eventually catch up? The parents would have been made anxious for no reason. Besides, if they are told that something appears to be wrong, there isn't much that can be done about brain injury anyway. We can't help them very much, so what can be achieved by confirming their fears?

However, in our experience, we have found that most parents are very realistic about their child's problems, and they want to know the truth. They don't want to be protected by false assurances, for their fears for their child cannot be this easily allayed.

If parents were listened to and their suspicions investigated, the treatment of brain injury would be more successful. Early detection is more likely to result in early intervention. In most cases, the child has a better chance of making good progress if the treatment is started while he is still young – in fact, the earlier it begins, the better.

Sometimes, even though the problem may be detected early, a wait and see approach is adopted in the hope that some spontaneous improvement may occur. There have been cases of natural recovery in these early years, since the brain of a young child is still in its dynamic growth period. The potential for self-repair in the brain seems greater at this time. But there are inherent risks with such an approach. It's all very well if the child does eventually catch up – the problem will have been alleviated without any unnecessary burden on the parents, and without the child having to undergo any type of therapy.

What happens though, if the child *doesn't* make significant improvement? Valuable treatment time will have been lost, and the child's condition may well have deteriorated. To ensure the best chance for progress, the parents – and the child – should not be denied the opportunity to try and put things right.

It may be said that parents could not deal with the emotional trauma of being told that there is something wrong with their child's brain, seeing that brain injury is thought to be a catastrophic condition. Certainly, if at the same time as they are told that their child is brain injured they are also informed that there is little hope of improvement, this diagnosis would have a daunting effect on any parent. Unfortunately, this is what sometimes happens today, and it makes many parents give up hope – even before they have started.

Instead, if parents were told there is evidence to suggest that brain injury may be helped with appropriate therapy, a much more positive attitude should prevail. This is not an offer of false hope, since no promises are given, and the evidence that it is based on is sufficient to suggest that brain injury is not necessarily a hopeless condition. Rather, it is an offer of realistic hope, for, without it, what chance has the child got?

* * *

But what of those parents who are still searching in vain for some-one who will listen to them? Those still knocking on door after door with the two questions they desperately want answered: 'What is wrong with our child? What can we do about it?'

Unfortunately, many haven't even got an answer to the first question yet.

Here is what one parent – Jenny Waddell of Melbourne, mother of nine-year-old Duncan – has to say about the frustration and heartbreak she went through knowing that something was wrong with her child, but being unable to convince anyone else:

Today, parents who discover that they have a child with brain injury have to fight hard to convince specialists of their belief, and *this is not fair*. The future road is tough enough without this added burden, and sometimes it becomes almost too much for parents to face.

But, it is these same parents who *must* quickly develop massive amounts of inner strength – the will of a tiger, and the unshakeable desire to help their child happily reach his or her full potential and achieve self-satisfaction in life.

The following is a step-by-step, frustration-by-frustration account of what I went through in trying to find some answers for my child:

In the beginning:

'Doctor, my newborn baby is so good – he never cries, he sleeps so well.'

At two months:

'Doctor, there is something wrong. My baby is too good. He never cries, he only wants to sleep, and he doesn't know me. You say I am imagining it.'

At three months:

'Doctor, there is definitely a problem with my baby, and I have sent him to a specialist as you suggested. Yes, he has ten fingers and ten toes. Why does everyone patronize me when I am in such a predicament?

Later:

'Doctor, I have been here many times. I am telling you there is a big problem. He doesn't play, he doesn't laugh, he hates to be held, he rocks in his cot and knocks his head against the wall. You say to move the cot from the wall. Fine, I will, but the wall is not the problem.'

Later:

'Doctor, I have reached the stage of total frustration and physical exhaustion. My child screams out loud for no reason, he never plays, he hates to be moved from his room. I have visited the specialist and yourself (not to mention the ear specialist when you thought Duncan might be deaf), so many times that I have lost track. And yet, my child is getting nowhere fast. Please help me to help my child. What is the matter with him? You suggest a psychiatrist'.

Later:

'Psychiatrist, you have been taking copious notes, and the many visits have not given you any indication as to the problem. I have been thinking of an alternative method of treatment, what is your opinion? Why are you horrified when the conventional methods have nothing to offer but sedatives and medicines? Now you tell me, after I decide to try another avenue, that my child is autistic and must be cared for by professional people who understand the problem. I *want* to understand! I love him and I am better equipped than all the professional people in the world to care for him, simply because I am his mother'.

CHAPTER THREE

The Labelling Syndrome

IF PARENTS of brain injured children wait long enough, they will eventually get the doctors to admit that something is wrong with their child. But what may have been a small problem when the parents first detected it within months of the child's birth, is likely to be more severe with the passing of time. For instance, if the problem is not medically diagnosed until the child is, say, fifteen months old, there is a strong possibility that he will be much further behind his peers than he was at two months – the age when his parents first knew that something was wrong.

Most therapists strongly advocate early detection followed by early intervention. For instance, Guilfoyle and associates state the case from a therapist's point of view: 'It is little wonder that therapists prefer to treat the newborn or young child, instead of being forced to wait until the child reaches school age. It is at this early age that the brain more than doubles its volume, and is probably the most plastic and the easiest to modify and to demonstrate significant changes due to therapeutic intervention.' [1]

In one sense, time is the enemy of brain injured children. If they are not developing at a normal rate, they slip further and further behind as time goes on. In this way, their condition actually gets worse.

Once the doctor admits there is a problem, parents breathe a sigh of relief thinking that at last something can be done. They expect to be given an explanation of what is wrong. After all, it has taken the doctors so long to recognize the problem, surely they have had enough time to determine exactly what it is. All the parents want is to know the nature of their child's condition, what caused it, and how it can be treated. To them, these are not unreasonable expectations.

However, they soon discover it is not that simple. For instance, in the beginning, all they may be told is that their child is 'developmentally delayed'. Yet they already know this – their child's slow development was the very reason why they have been concerned for so long. So the parents press for more information. Depending on the child's specific problems, terms such as 'cerebral palsy' and 'mental retardation' may eventually be used. These labels often come as a great shock to the parents, as they may have always imagined that these conditions were permanent, and associated with people in wheelchairs or in mental institutions.

The doctor may now tell them that, historically, these children have not made very much progress. Therefore, while not completely giving up on their child, they should realize that they can't hope for much improvement. The best thing they can do is to gradually get used to the idea that their child will never be normal.

With such news, the parents can sink even further into despair. Until then they may have been confident that they would be able to do something about their child's problem. To be told otherwise in such definite terms is devastating for them.

Some parents remain determined to do all they can to help their child, despite the gloomy picture that has been presented, and this strong will carries them through the empty and depressing times ahead. Sadly, for others, the doctor's message takes the wind out of their sails. They never really recover. All hope is gone, never to return.

* * *

For those able to carry on, the first move is to discover the meaning of the names given to describe their child's condition. If their child has been labelled as 'cerebral palsy', the doctor may have told them that this is the name given to describe a condition in which the child's movement is hindered, or prevented, by abnormal muscle tone. But this is already obvious to them. They had realized long ago that the reason their child couldn't reach out was because his arms were too stiff, and he couldn't crawl on his tummy because he wasn't able to bend and straighten his legs properly. To call this 'cerebral palsy' sounds very technical, but it doesn't give them any new information about their child. It does not tell them what caused the problem, or how it could be treated, and probably they know that there is no such disease as 'cerebral palsy', that it isn't something you catch like a virus. The same confusion would also arise if the parents were told that their child was suffering from 'mental retardation', for this label is as unclear as 'cerebral palsy' in terms of telling the parents what caused the problem and how it could be treated.

In fact, both cerebral palsy and mental retardation are just symptomatic descriptions of the child's condition. To the child's parents, this is of no real help, for they need to know about the cause rather than the symptoms, since it seems obvious to them that any treatment should be directed at the cause of the problem. They know that when you have an infection, you treat the cause by taking medication that fights the infection, instead of just taking pain killers to relieve the symptoms. They naturally expect that this same principle would apply to their child's problem.

Most medical conditions are diagnosed and treated according to the cause. If you had an acute pain in your side and suspected that this was caused by appendicitis, you would want to find a doctor who would investigate your suspicion, and then treat the cause of the problem accordingly.

But imagine if you were treated by someone who only dealt with the symptoms of illness. His diagnosis of your complaint would be 'acute lower abdominal pain', as this accurately describes the symptoms you were suffering. The subsequent treatment would be concerned only with relieving your symptom – the pain – and initially, it would appear to be successful. But if the infection got worse, as it may do without proper treatment, the pain would increase and you would have to take more and more of the pain-killing medication. If the cause of the pain continued to be ignored, the infection could spread, causing serious problems, and possibly even resulting in death.

Fortunately, this type of medicine is rarely practised these days. In most circumstances, the diagnosis is made according to the cause, and it is the cause that is treated. 'Appendicitis' tells you that the pain is due to an inflamed and infected appendix, and this is what is treated.

However, as parents of brain injured children often discover, not all medical diagnosis and treatment is cause-related. Many of the labels that their children are given are simply labels that describe the symptoms. As well, like pain killers for appendicitis, much of the treatment given is directed at the symptoms rather than the cause. Take mental retardation for example: the goal of the treatment for these children seems to be concerned with doing the best you can within the confines of their apparently limited potential. This treatment will involve things such as teaching basic learning skills, independence, and social awareness. Unfortunately, this doesn't seem to be enough, since even though these children may show improvement, in almost all cases they still remain mentally retarded to some degree.

The problem is that no real attempt is made to try and treat the underlying cause of the mental retardation. Instead, treatment is directed at improving the symptoms as much as possible – to do the best with what you have got, rather than changing what you've got.

* * *

Historically, symptomatic labelling of problems related to brain injury has always been present, although the labels have gradually changed. For instance, eighty years ago, a mentally retarded person was often referred to as either an idiot, imbecile, or moron, depending on the severity of his problem. Such people were locked away in mental institutions, and were considered to be incurable and somewhat inhuman.

These labels have evolved over the years to keep pace with changing social attitudes, so as to move away from the implied hopelessness of these early labels. The words idiot, imbecile and moron became emotionally charged, so eventually the term 'mental retardation' was introduced. In the beginning, this was quite acceptable, but with time, it too became inappropriate.

'Mental retardation' had outlived its day, so once again it was time to invent a new label. Today, such nice terms as 'special' and 'exceptional' are used. This makes it sound as if it's not really too bad to be mentally retarded, but parents are not fooled by such semantic games.

Unfortunately, the medical profession is sometimes so intent on finding a label to put on a child's condition, that more effort is put into diagnosis than into treatment. Many cases of brain injury are complex, often without any apparent cause, and frequently manifesting in many different symptoms. Thus, labelling is extremely difficult if the symptoms are the only criteria used. In such situations children can go through months and months of testing, seeing many different doctors, and in the final analysis, the parents are still as confused as to the real nature of their child's condition. Often, no treatment is suggested until a clear diagnosis is made, so valuable therapy time is lost.

When a child is given a label, he is usually stuck with it for the rest of his life. If such labels get caught up in the bureaucracy that seems to surround most social welfare systems, confusion is usually the end result. For example, take the following case as described in this excerpt from a letter concerning the future welfare of a brain injured child. Don't worry if you find it very confusing, we did too!

The report is that the EEG was abnormal, and associated with her general delay in development, the neurologist has classified her as 'cerebral palsy'. We have been carrying her in our clinic as a child with 'developmental delay', but now she is three years of age, she needs to be classified as 'severe cerebral palsy' or 'severe developmental delay', in order to receive nursery school benefits.

The services would be the same until this September; however, by then, it would be wise to classify her as either 'severe cerebral palsy' or 'severe developmental delay'. Her absence of a motor deficit is so pronounced, because of her ability to walk etc., that I do not think she could be classified as 'severe cerebral palsy'. However, her cognitive development [understanding] is sufficiently delayed that she could be classified as 'severe brain damage', representing herself by 'severe developmental retardation'. Her mother seems very receptive and understanding of this, and I think it might be the kind of thing she could think about. We will be very willing to reclassify her in this area to receive compensation to benefit the child's program.

Such an example typifies what can go wrong if symptomatic labels are used. Perhaps it is best summed up by the slogan we once saw on a protest-button: *Label Jars, not People.*

CHAPTER FOUR

'Brain Injury' – More Than Just Another Label

PROFESSOR Sir John Eccles, Nobel Prize-winning Australian neurophysiologist, sums up the importance of the human brain with these simple words: 'The brain literally gives us everything. It gives us the whole wonder of our existence, our individual conscious existence, everything that we are – our own self and personality'.[1]

Since the role of the brain is so significant, there can be drastic consequences if it is injured in any way. It is brain injury that is responsible for many of the developmental problems that occur in children. Cerebral palsy is a symptom of brain injury; so too is mental retardation, as are some cases of developmental delay, speech and learning problems, autism, intellectual handicap. All of these can be the result of some kind of injury to the brain.

The type of problem that manifests is dependent on the nature and extent of the injury that has occurred. In cases of severe injury, many different problems exist, since different parts of the brain have been affected. If each of these problems is looked at in isolation, a true picture of the child's overall problem cannot be gained. For instance, some two-year-old children have been given as many as five different labels – their medical reports may describe the child as suffering from cerebral palsy, mental retardation, developmental delay, ataxia, and cortical blindness. Is it that these children have five different problems requiring five different labels? Or is it that they have one problem – brain injury – that has led to these five different symptoms?

'Brain injury' is the appropriate diagnosis to use when the problem stems from an injury to the brain, as it very clearly recognizes the *cause* of the disorder. The symptomatic labels may be of some value if they are used in conjunction with the diagnosis of brain injury, as they would then describe the type of brain injury that has occurred. But used in isolation, they do nothing more than describe the symptoms.

As obvious as it may seem, the term 'brain injury' is not often used as a diagnosis, especially in the case of younger children. In fact, there seems to be something of a professional reluctance to use these words. This is probably because many people think that brain injury is a condition from which little recovery can be made. If this were true, then the use of symptomatic labels would be completely justified. They would be less daunting than a diagnosis that immediately branded a child as 'hopeless'. But since we believe that brain injury *can* be treated, often quite successfully, we feel that there is no reason to hide the truth behind protective labels.

Before 'brain injury' can be used universally as a diagnosis, the pessimism and confusion that still exists regarding its use needs to be cleared up. If parents reviewed the medical literature on this subject, they would probably end up more puzzled than they were before they started. For instance, if we look more closely at the book quoted from at the start of this chapter, completely contrasting opinions are given at its beginning and end.

In the foreword, Professor John Eccles states: 'Let us now examine the post-natal stage of a child with brain damage. Neurogenesis (the growth of new brain cells) is virtually complete and no more structural development is possible after birth. It might be said, then, that brain damage cannot be treated; that after birth the brain cannot make up for deficiencies.

This is a misunderstanding. Although a child is born with a damaged brain, or a deficient brain, there is an immense potential that awaits realization.' However, at the end of the book, the editor, Perry Black, has this to say in the epilogue: 'While all behaviour, as well as intellectual and neurological functions must, in the last analysis, have their origins in the brain, terms such as minimal brain dysfunction implies structural damage and hence irreversibility and hopelessness.'

Confusion indeed, underlying the great need for a better understanding of brain injury, of the use of 'brain injury' as a diagnosis, and of the potential for recovery of function after injury to the brain, which, according to Eccles, 'awaits realization'.

What is actually meant by the term 'brain injury', and how can it be caused? Brain injury occurs when brain cells are destroyed, or prevented from developing normally, by some kind of insult to the brain, either at the time of conception, during the pregnancy, around the time of birth, or any time after birth.

At the time of conception, an error in the genetic blueprint contained within the egg or sperm can result in a number of chromosome abnormalities that can affect the brain of the child (such as Down's Syndrome). Excessive alcohol intake by either or both parents before conception, or by the mother during the pregnancy, can have a damaging effect on the foetal brain.[2]

During the pregnancy, there are many things that could go wrong which may cause injury to the developing brain. The mother without immunity may be exposed to a virus such as rubella, she may be in very poor health, have a low quality diet, she may suffer severe emotional stress, or have a serious fall or accident.

Around the time of birth, the brain of the baby may be adversely affected by things such as extreme prematurity or postmaturity, a prolonged or precipitous labour, or some kind of delivery complication.

After birth, the newborn could have trouble maintaining independent respiration, resulting in short periods without oxygen that could be detrimental to the brain. Illnesses that the child may contract, such as meningitis and encephalitis, could also have a drastic effect. Traumatic insults to the brain could occur at any time during childhood or adulthood, and result in brain injury. Such traumas as near drownings, electric shock, poisoning, drug overdoses, and head injuries from car, motorbike, or sporting accidents might be responsible.

These are just some of the things that could cause brain injury. However, it needs to be emphasized that a person can suffer from any one of the traumas mentioned and still remain perfectly normal. Even if brain injury is caused, it may not be severe enough to result in any problems becoming evident.

Table 3 details the way that mental retardation can occur. Since mental retardation is usually a symptom of brain injury, this table gives a good indication of the causes of brain injury.

The different symptoms of brain injury can be viewed as belonging to an overall continuum of neurological development, as described in Table 4.

Every person, brain injured or normal, is on this continuum. Where they are is determined by the amount of brain injury that has occurred (pathology), and the quality and quantity of environmental

Table 3: Causes of 5,200 cases of mental retardation

World Health Organization classifications	Examples	%
Infections and intoxications	Meningitis, encephalitis	7.4
Trauma or physical agents	Head injuries, drownings	10.17
Disorders of metabolism, growth or diet	PKU, thyroid deficiency	3.83
Gross brain diseases	Tumours, cancers, etc	2.69
Unknown prenatal influences	Unknown	16.4
Chromosome abnormalities	Down's syndrome	17.96
Prematurity	O_2 lack, immature brain	4.73
Psychiatric disorders	Schizophrenia, autism	1.94
Environmental disorders	Lack of stimulation and movement	1.9
Other and unspecified	—	32.96

Based on a report from New South Wales Anti-Discrimination Board publication; *Discrimination and Intellectual Handicap*, N.S.W. Government publication, 1981.

stimulation they have been exposed to (neurological environment).

For normal people, who have obviously suffered very little pathology, their place on the continuum is largely dependent on the neurological environment that they have been in, especially in the early years of life. For brain injured children, it is a combination of both pathology and environment. The greater the pathology and the poorer the neurological environment, the greater the neurological dysfunction. The better the neurological environment and any improvement in the pathology, the better the neurological organization.

Although the symptoms of brain injury are extremely varied, they are all, in effect, different degrees of the same problem. All the levels of the continuum are related, as they represent the varying degrees of brain injury. You can move up and down this continuum, because of this relationship. If a brain injured child is at a particular level, it doesn't necessarily mean that he will stay there.

For instance, if he begins to make progress, he will move up the continuum, level by level. In recovery from coma, a child usually does not suddenly wake up and resume his normal life. Instead, the return of function is a gradual process. The coma progressively lightens until the child responds to environmental stimuli – at this

Continuum of neurological development

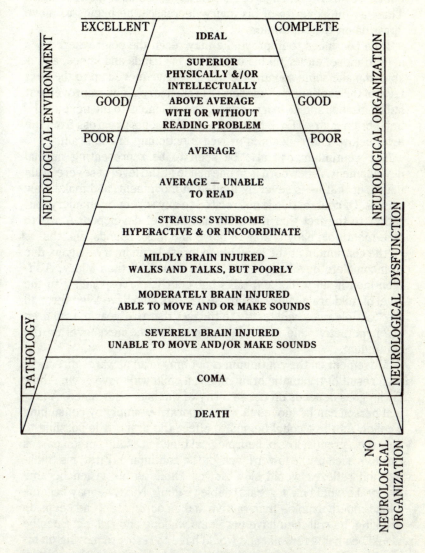

Table 4: Continuum of Neurological Development
© 1980, Sandler-Brown Consultants, Willow Grove, Pa., U.S.A.

point he is no longer in coma. However, he may still be unable to move or make sounds as a result of the continuing effects of the brain injury. He has now moved up to the next level of the continuum – 'severely brain injured, unable to move and/or make sounds'. Thus, as the severity of his injury decreases, he begins to move upwards on the continuum.

If he continues to improve, he may reach the point where he is able to move, either on his tummy or his hands and knees, and is able to make some sounds. He will now have moved up to the next level of the continuum – 'moderate brain injury'. If his improvement still continues and he learns to walk, he will move to the next level – 'mild brain injury'. Each higher level represents progress from the level below, and reflects improved functioning of the brain.

The continuum can also be seen to be representing normal development. A newborn is in one sense at the level of severe brain injury, in that he is severely limited in movement, and makes few sounds. Of course, this is not related to any sort of brain injury, but rather to the fact that the brain has not yet developed. A six- to nine-month-old baby is able to move and make sounds, and thus is on the continuum at the level of moderate brain injury – again, due to incomplete development of the brain rather than injury. A fifteen-month-old walks and talks but poorly, corresponding to the level of mild brain injury. All those parents who have lived through the 'terrible twos' will testify to the fact that two-year-old children are hyperactive and incoordinate, just like the next level on the continuum.

Movement on the continuum is not only in an upwards direction. As a result of traumatic brain injury, a child will move down – how far he goes depends on the severity of the injury sustained. A normal person can be moved down temporarily, simply by consuming alcohol. As the alcohol begins to affect the brain, it is possible to observe a gradual loss of neurological function as the person passes through each of the lower levels of the continuum. First, his thinking and reflexes would slow down. Then, as his vision became blurry, he would have great trouble reading. Next, he may become a loud-mouth drunk – hyperactive and incoordinate. If he keeps on drinking, he will then have problems walking and talking. Soon he would be unable to walk, and would have to resort to moving on his hands and knees, making unintelligible sounds. With further alcohol consumption, he'd soon be fast asleep – unable to move or make sounds. If further alcohol was put into his body, he could pass into a coma, and could even die. Thus, in the space of three to four hours, someone could move from near the top of the continuum right down to the bottom.

Brain growth is a dynamic process. Just because a brain injured child is at a specific level on the continuum does not mean this is where he has to stay. The objective with every child should be to move them upwards from their present level.

But how can this be done? Isn't the brain supposed to be an organ incapable of self-repair? What is the point of diagnosing according to the cause, if the cause cannot be treated? Can the brain's efficiency be improved?

The next section of this book attempts to answer some of these questions. Evidence will be given to show that the brain, rather than being unable to compensate after injury, is in fact a very dynamic organ with a previously unrecognized ability for repair and recovery. We think that you will be amazed and excited when you discover the potential that lies within the human brain.

Section II
The Potential within the Brain

CHAPTER FIVE

The World's Most Amazing Computer

AS THE 21st century approaches, the world is becoming more and more technologically orientated. In this 'Computer Age', ideas that seemed futuristic just ten years ago are now an everyday reality, for the computer is rapidly taking over industry and entering the domestic scene.

As we marvel at what computers can achieve, there is a tendency to forget about the original computer – the human brain. Since the workings of the brain remain one of life's greatest mysteries, its abilities tend to be under-estimated. In fact, the 'silicon chip generation' may tell you that the computers of today supersede the brain. But, as amazing as computers may be, they still cannot compare.

Rockets can be launched into outer space and can be programmed to send back photographs of distant planets, astronauts can be sent to the moon and back and the most complex computer systems imaginable can be constructed. Yet, despite years and years of research, scientists still are unsure about the precise way in which the human brain works. In fact, when writing about the brain, the biggest difficulty occurs in trying to report concrete information. Much of the data is based on hypotheses only. Such data, although well informed, cannot be completely substantiated. There is also disagreement amongst scientists, and it is very frustrating to read one interpretation of a particular aspect of brain function, only to have it contradicted in the next book that one picks up.

However, one fact is certain, the working parts that exist in the human brain are so vast in number as to be virtually beyond comprehension. In fact, this is the very essence of the problem. The brain, being so amazingly complex and intricate in design, defies accurate scientific description.

The number of working parts in the brain, and the tremendous amount of organization and control required to keep everything running smoothly, makes even the most advanced computer seem primitive. Taking a look at some facts and figures gives an idea of the enormity of the brain, but these are only estimates, and conflicting reports in other publications may be found. Still, they serve to represent the amazing complexity that exists.

According to Nauta[1], an American neuroanatomist, the number of neurons (the nerve cell in the brain that is responsible for transmitting impulses) thought to be in the human central nervous system is usually estimated at around 10^{10}, or 100,000,000,000. But Nauta feels that this figure may be a modest estimate, and he suggests that the number may be as high as 10^{11}, or even 10^{12}.

Each neuron forms an enormous number of connections with other neurons. Barr[2] states that between 1,000 and 100,000 (10,000 on average) synapses can be found on a single nerve cell body and its processes (a synapse is the connection point between one neuron and another). Granit[3] puts this average number at 30,000. This results in an almost incalculable number of different ways that messages can be relayed in the brain. Buzan[4] has estimated that the number of possible interconnections within the human brain is 10^{800}.

One of the most puzzling aspects of the way the brain operates is the manner in which it seems to use only a small proportion of the total number of neurons available. For instance, a surprisingly tiny number act as motor neurons – the cells that control movement. Nauta (see note 1 above) estimates that there cannot be more than two or three million used for this specific purpose. According to Nauta: 'this is a disconcertingly small number in view of the fact that only through motor neurons can the workings of the nervous system find expression in movement'.

If this figure is true (Nauta does not explain how he arrived at his calculation), then why are so many neurons present when only a small number are used specifically for motor function? Nauta attempts to explain this by referring to what he calls the 'great intermediate net' – neurons that are neither sensory nor motor, but act as go-betweens along the path of sensory-to-motor transfer of impulses.

The work of Jacobson, published in 1978 (and earlier with Hirsch in 1975)[5,6], offers a further explanation. He states that there appear to be two main classes of neurons – Class I (or principal) neurons, and Class II neurons. These two different neurons vary in their structure, and also in the way that they grow. Class I neurons form and develop at an early stage of embryonic growth. They make the primary connections in the brain, so their functions need to be specified early on. This means that their functions are fixed and cannot be modified later. These neurons complete their development at a time when the embryo is still largely protected from the environment.

The Class II neurons are formed at a later stage of embryonic growth. Their development also occurs later, often postnatally – therefore, they are more exposed to environmental influence. These neurons are smaller and unspecified, and they have the ability to be modified. Jacobson suggests that it is these cells which may be responsive to environmental influences, and thus responsible for the plastic or modifiable aspects of behaviour (see note 5 above). According to Granit (see note 3 above), they require stimulation for their development, and for the maintenance of their function.

Jacobson refers to these Class II neurons as 'interneurons' (see note 5 above) – this is perhaps the same as Nauta's 'great intermediate net' (see note 1 above). Granit states that the cortex is primarily an expansion of unspecified interneurons, enormous in number, and open to environmental modifications (see note 3 above). Nauta's figure regarding the small number of motor neurons in the cortex certainly supports this concept (see note 1 above). If there is such a small number of motor neurons, there must be a vast number of unspecified cortical cells.

Common sense dictates that there must be some kind of compensation system existing in the human brain. It is unlikely that such an amazingly sophisticated piece of machinery could have a major flaw in its design – the inability to grow new cells to replace destroyed ones – without having an alternate system by which the recovery of function could occur. Other systems in the body use the growth of new cells as an effective means of self-repair. For instance, this happens with the skin and the liver.

Evidence that some kind of compensation system does exist is the fact that recovery of function after brain injury can and does occur, sometimes quite spontaneously – despite the brain's inability to grow new cells. Such recovery can only happen if other cells somehow take over the functions of the destroyed cells. Luria, a famous Russian psychologist, and his associates confirm this viewpoint when they state: 'the restoration of function follows a different road in cases where the disturbance is based on an irreversible destruction of nerve cells. In this case, restoration of function in its original form is impossible. The only way left is to reconstruct the disturbed function to include intact nerve cells in its restoration, to transfer it to another intact neural apparatus, and sometimes to modify its psychophysiological composition radically, so that the original task is performed by new methods and by means of a completely new neural organization'.[7]

Thus, to compensate for the absence of a repair system that utilizes new cell growth, it seems that the brain does have an alternate system. It appears able to somehow arrange for the cells unaffected by the injury to take over from the destroyed ones. This prevents loss of function following a very mild injury, and helps to prevent complete devastation following a major insult to the brain. It also enables the gradual recovery of function that can occur following brain injury.

If such a system does exist, then a vast network of adaptable, non-specific neurons must be present. The Class II neurons which comprise most of the cortex of the brain appear ideally suited for this purpose. Indeed, it seems that this is one of the roles they play in the brain.

We now need to look at how this and other systems can be utilized to facilitate recovery of function following brain injury.

CHAPTER SIX

The Adaptability of the Human Brain

WE ARE only beginning to appreciate just how adaptable is the human brain. No longer can it be thought of as a hard-wired system with little ability for self-repair. Rather, as the evidence in this chapter will show, it has an enormous potential for recovery of function following injury. For instance, we can take a look at what scientists who have spent most of their lives studying the brain have to say.

Granit[1] describes the brain as having 'an incredible degree of adaptability as yet by no means fully explored'. Brodal[2] says: 'We may consider the brain as consisting of a multitude of small units, each with its particular morphological (and presumably functional) features. These units collaborate by way of an immensely rich, complicated and differentiated network of connections, which are precisely and specifically organized. The anatomical possibilities for (more or less direct) co-operation between various parts of the brain must be almost unlimited'.

This adaptability of the brain is often referred to as its 'plasticity'. Bach-y-Rita[3] states that: 'Brain plasticity refers to the adaptive capacities of the central nervous system – its ability to modify its own structural organization and functioning. It is an adaptive response to functional demand . . . plasticity permits enduring functional changes to take place.'

In the preface to a recent (1981) book concerning neuronal plasticity, the editors Flohr and Precht[4] write: 'Sensorimotor systems are not rigidly wired, predetermined networks, but rather highly plastic structures that learn and modify their entire performance in response to changes in external or internal conditions. Lesions or distortions of the system's input, which initially cause a functional disorganization, induce an active reorganization which often leads to a recovery of function. Examples of lesion-induced neural plasticity have been known for some hundred years; however, an awareness of their value as research tools is relatively new. This current interest is a consequence of rapidly changing ideas concerning the nature of CNS (central nervous system) organization. Out of these, concepts are emerging which describe neural nets as modifiable, highly dynamic, self-organizing structures.'

Scientists have studied the different ways that the brain can adapt following injury, and they have developed various theories. We will now take a look at some of these.

1 Spare capacity and reorganization

Most studies concerning recovery of function following brain injury have been done with animals, simply because the final part of the study has often required removal of the brain to examine the damaged areas. Some people say that the results of these animal studies cannot be directly applied to humans, but the scientists involved are adamant that their work sheds a great deal of light on how the human brain functions.

However, although vital information can be gained from animal studies, it is obvious that the evidence is more conclusive if the studies involve human beings. In this respect, there are a great many examples of remarkable recovery of function occurring in humans following brain injury. For instance, Bach-y-Rita (see note 3 above) describes the case of his father who suffered a stroke at the age of sixty-five. He made an almost complete recovery, and he returned to his work as a college professor three years later and led an active life until he died at seventy-two, of a heart attack while on a mountain hiking trip. By way of an autopsy, it was possible to see what damage had been caused to his brain at the time of the stroke. In fact, he had incurred a massive injury, for in the corticospinal pathways of the lower brain-stem and spinal cord, only 3 per cent of the nerve fibres that were capable of transferring information in the brain remained intact. Yet, despite such a small part of the brain being undamaged, he was able to make full recovery. In attempting to explain this phenomenon, Bach-y-Rita suggests the functional recovery that occurred is evidence of a high level of plasticity, and that the 3 per cent of remaining normal fibres possibly served as the basis for this reorganization.

The work of Lorber[5] provides another startling example of how the human brain can adapt. His research concerned patients suffering from spina bifida, a congenital condition in which the spinal column of the developing foetus fails to close completely, resulting in symptoms ranging from weak muscles and poor skin sensation to paralysis of the legs and loss of bladder control.

One of the complications that can be associated with spina bifida is a condition known as 'hydrocephalus', an abnormal collection of cerebro-spinal fluid in the brain. With this excess of fluid, the ventricles (the fluid reserves in the brain) expand. This increase in the ventricle size can be damaging to the brain, as the enlarged ventricles can impinge on brain cells and destroy them. Thus, severe cases of hydrocephalus can decrease the amount of brain tissue available, resulting in intellectual and physical disabilities.

Professor Lorber studied 600 spina bifida patients who had the added complication of hydrocephalus. He did brain scans on each of these patients to determine the amount of fluid accumulation, and he then compared these to the scans of normal brains. Based on this comparison, the 600 patients were divided into the following four categories:

1: those with minimally enlarged ventricles
2: ventricle expansion equal to 50-70% of the cranium
3: ventricle expansion equal to 70-90% of the cranium
4: ventricle expansion greater than 90% of the cranium

Looking at the fourth category, it is amazing that anyone survived such a massive insult to the brain, and it is not surprising that some of these people had severe neurological problems. But, as incredible as it may seem, some were functioning quite well. Lorber found that 50 per cent of those in this category had IQ scores of greater than 100! Thus, despite such an enormous loss of brain tissue, these people were still able to function at a normal intellectual level.

In one particularly dramatic case, a university student was referred to Lorber because his head seemed slightly larger than normal. A subsquent brain scan showed a gigantic fluid accumulation – instead of a normal 4.5 cm depth of cortical tissue between the ventricles and the outer layer of the cortex, there was only a thin layer of brain tissue measuring barely a millimetre. Despite having such a minute amount of brain available, the student had an IQ of 126, a first-class honours degree in mathematics, and was socially quite normal!

It is little wonder that the article describing Lorber's findings was provocatively titled 'Is your brain really necessary?', for it certainly highlights an almost incredible degree of human brain adaptation?

Lorber's findings are not unique, for according to Wall (see note 5), there are scores of similar accounts in medical literature. For instance, Glees[6] studied humans who had undergone hemispherectomies, the surgical removal of parts of one hemisphere of the brain. This operation leads to a loss of brain tissue varying from 170 to 300 grams. Despite such extensive removal of brain tissue, the patients still functioned quite well. This was proof to Glees of 'the remarkable ability of the remaining brain tissue for reorganization and the achievement of useful function for the total organism'.

How is it that normal or near-normal function can continue when so much destruction of the brain occurs? According to Lorber (see note 5 above), this suggests there must be a tremendous amount of spare capacity or redundancy in the brain, resulting in the brain being able to utilize some cells unaffected by injury, in an attempt to restore function. Blakemore states that spare capacity is an important quality of the human brain. He says: 'The brain frequently has to cope with minor lesions, and it is crucial that it can overcome these radily.' He believes that this can occur by reorganization of brain tissue, and by reallocation of function. (See note 5 above.)

This process of reorganization seems to be critical to the successful utilization of the spare capacity of the brain. Luria[7] feels that adaptation occurs following injury as a result of the internal reorganization of the parts of the brain unaffected by the damage. As well, the destroyed area can be replaced by another which is still intact, thereby including into the functional system areas that are able to compensate, in one form or another, for the lost element. Luria shows how this can happen by referring to the process of normal development – during the developmental process, the brain matures and higher cortical areas take control. This results in an intensive reorganization of the brain, with the same task being performed by completely different means.

Sameroff and Chandler[8] also hold a similar view of normal development. They view normal brain growth as being a succession of 'qualitative reorganizations', each of which may incorporate adjustments to function. These adjustments may overcome the effects of insult, thereby redirecting development toward a normal level.

In the case of normal development, the growth or virtual reorganization of the brain occurs over an extended period of time. Thus, it would seem logical that if reorganization was to occur following brain injury, this, too, would be a long-term process. As well, according to Luria, such reorganization is largely dependent on long and specialized training (see note 7 above).

·It is significant that most of Lorber's spina bifida patients who retained normal function in certain areas, had suffered a slowly developing hydrocephalus (see note 5 above). In spina bifida-related hydrocephalus, there is a slow build-up of fluid over many years. In situations where the build-up of fluid occurs suddenly, such as after severe head injury, a great deal of damage and subsequent loss of function can be caused by this fluid increase.

Time is the critical factor here. If the increase in fluid is sudden, there seems to be a greater loss of function than if a gradual increase occurs. Could it be that, with time, the brain has the chance to reorganize and adapt? There seems to be evidence to suggest that this is in fact what does happen.

Stein and Lewis[9] and Stein and Schultze[10] have studied the effects of time on the restoration of function in rats following brain injury. Two groups of rats were subjected to identical amounts of brain injury, in exactly the same brain area. The only difference was that the injury in one group was created in two or more stages, with several weeks interval between each stage. The other group received the injury all at once.

During the testing period, the two groups were given the same amount of recovery time, and they were placed in the same environment. At the end of the study, the scientists reported that the rats which received their injury in stages, performed significantly better than those in the other group.

In attempting to explain this difference in performance, the scientists said that the better function of the rats injured over several stages did not necessarily reflect healing of the injured part of the brain. Rather, it possibly represented the activation of an alternate system.

They proposed that the function of some of the brain structures may have been taken over by undamaged tissue in the situations where the damage was inflicted gradually. Thus, by the time the second and subsequent injuries were created, there may have been a transfer of function – the result of the reorganization of undamaged tissue around the injured site. Therefore, the effects of the later injuries were reduced.

A close examination of these rats' brains revealed that there was no growth of new brain cells, so the improved function must have been as a result of the utilization of existing tissue. When the time was made available for reorganization to occur, this is exactly what happened.

Curiously enough, the same thing appears to have happened with Lorber's spina bifida patients. Looking at the comparative effects of sudden and gradual hydrocephalus, patients have a much better chance of functioning well if the increase in fluid occurs gradually. It appears that the patient can cope with this loss of brain cells by the process of continual reorganization – providing that the time is available for this to occur.

It may well be that in these cases, it is not so much a question of how many brain cells are available or how many have been destroyed, but rather how well the brain is organized to use what is there.

The brains of Lorber's spina bifida patients in the fourth category must have become extremely well organized – for how else could these people perform so well, given that they only have such a tiny amount of brain tissue available? (See note 5 above.)

2 Redundancy

Closely related to the theory of reorganization of the brain following injury is the concept of 'redundancy'. This refers to the way that the brain seems to have a system of duplicated pathways for controlling the same function. This means that if one pathway is damaged or destroyed, the possibility exists that one of the duplicated pathways may take over.

According to Granit: 'Everywhere one finds important functions secured by a redundancy of pathways, and also by a multiplicity of mechanisms capable of producing the same end effect.' In looking at why redundancy occurs, Granit states: 'The brain has to cope with both basic predictability and Nature's capriciousness. This is done by having strictly designed pathways on one hand, and an immense multiplication of possibilities on the other. This immense multiplication is reminiscent of the apparent wastefulness of plants and animals in producing seeds, sperm and eggs, but is necessary to ensure the continued adaptation of the species' (see note 1 above).

In humans, the normal development of the brain seems to result in a certain degree of redundancy. Granit feels that as the brain matures, some circuits become dominant while others appear to be relegated to a recessive role. Either that or they are over-ridden and in turn controlled in part by newer pathways. Ayers[11] refers to the control exerted by the higher parts of the brain as being additional, but not substitute, control. She says: 'As the nervous system evolved to meet the expanding needs of existence, the newer structures tended to duplicate older structures and functions, and improve on them rather than to devise different functions. Nature, like some people, hesitates to throw anything away; instead, it will modify the function of the older structure. Thus the same kinds of functions are repeated at several levels of the brain. The higher levels, as they developed, also remained dependent upon the lower structures.'

Moore[12] explains what happens to the lower brain levels as the higher parts take over: 'As higher level functions develop, the older pathways that once performed a patterned response are no longer vital for carrying out a particular activity pattern. This is not to say that these older routes die out or fade away. They remain, and function in the normal individual in maintaining the overall integrity of the nervous system. However, they function in a minor way in comparison to the newer pathways . . .'

According to Moore, these redundant levels may be utilized following an injury that destroys parts of the higher centres: 'When higher functions are lost or damaged due to brain injury, the older, once-utilized, recessive or alternate routes remain. If these can be tapped or strengthened – by using them in the same way, or in a manner similar to the way they were originally used – then these older pathways may constitute viable "alternate potentials" through which functional alternatives may be gained.'

3 Response at a cellular level

Once it was realized that it was impossible for new cells to grow following brain cell destruction, attention was directed towards trying to discover how the surrounding cells, unaffected by the injury, respond. This was because it was thought that these were the cells responsible for any restoration of function that did occur.

It was through the work of Lui and Chambers[13] in 1958 that the first evidence of brain cell adaptation was seen under the microscope. The introduction of the electron microscope around this time enabled the scientists to study in finer detail the minute world of the nerve connections in the brain.

After creating injury in the brain of a rat, Lui and Chambers discovered that the undamaged axons (the transmitting 'wires' coming from the nerve cell that relays messages to other cells) in the vicinity of the damaged area attempted to rewire what had been lost through injury. They did this by sending out new connections, or 'sprouts', as Lui and Chambers described them. They called this phenomenon 'collateral sprouting', and it was thought that this was the means by which the brain was attempting to compensate for its inability to grow new brain cells.

This startling discovery naturally created a great deal of excitement in the scientific world. Additional studies were done to test Lui and Chambers' work, and these reinforced the original findings.[14,15,16] The fact that collateral sprouting does occur is now beyond dispute. But just when and why it occurs, and in what parts of the brain, is still not clearly understood.

Some studies show that collateral sprouting can occur to a much greater extent than was first realized. For instance, a 1976 study by Matthews[17] showed that after an injury destroyed all but 14 per cent of the connections in a specific area of a rat's brain, up to 80 per cent of the original connections were restored in 280 days – presumably by the process of collateral sprouting.

There is still a great deal of dispute as to how much function can be derived from the new connections established by the collateral sprouting. Some studies suggest that no functional use can be achieved by these new connections, while others even feel that the new pathways can have an adverse effect in some situations.[18,19,20] There are others who are just as adamant that the rewiring results in permanent functional connections.[21]

Putting aside for the moment the argument concerning its effectiveness, just the fact that collateral sprouting does occur is indisputable evidence that the brain attempts, at a cellular level, to restore function following injury.

According to Wall[22], there are other ways by which the remaining brain cells may attempt to compensate after injury. For instance, he says that nerve cells show a type of homeostasis – an inbuilt system designed to maintain the proper equilibrium within the brain. By this means, the remaining nerve cells can become more excitable, thereby increasing their ability to receive information. St James-Roberts[23] refers to this process as 'denervation supersensitivity'.

Wall proposes another type of cellular adaptation, which is really a form of redundancy: '. . . there are large numbers of normally ineffective nerve connections which may become active if the dominant inputs are put out of action. It is proposed that the connections laid down in the embryo are more diffuse than those actually used in the adult brain. The stages of maturation partly involve destruction of the "incorrect" connections, and partly their suppression. If some nervous connections are destroyed in the adult, suppressed connections may become de-repressed. This process is not necessarily a good thing, for the substituted connections may bring in nonsense information which the recovering nervous system cannot handle'.

Wall clearly summarizes how collateral sprouting and redundancy contribute to the recovery of function: 'Sprouting and the unmasking of ineffective connections offers the possibility of new connections after brain damage, but we need to know much more about these processes so that we can guide them to useful ends rather than towards further disorganization' (see note 22 above).

4 Environmental effects

It has been known for some time that increased environmental stimulation usually results in improved performance in animals and humans. Since the 1950s, improved scientific techniques have allowed researchers to demonstrate that this stimulation directly affects the brain cells, thereby showing that the effect goes beyond simply achieving better function.

Studies in this area fall into three major categories: the effects of increased environmental stimulation on normal animals; the effects of decreased stimulation; and, most importantly, the question of whether or not increased stimulation has any effect on recovery of function following brain injury.

i Environmental enrichment

Many studies, including those of Rosenzweig[24] and Goldman[25], show that increased environmental stimulation results in improved performance. Of greater interest are the studies that demonstrate that not only does increased stimulation produce increased abilities, it actually increases brain growth. In these particular studies[26,27,28,29], rats were put into three different environments for the exact same period of time. The environments were varied according to the amount of stimulation they offered – either normal, deprived or enriched.

At the end of the study period, the rats were tested and, as expected, those that had been in the enriched environment performed significantly better than those in the other two groups. When the rats were sacrificed and their brains studied, a startling revelation was made. Without exception, the rats which had been living in the enriched world had brains that were bigger in weight and dimension, along with increased chemical activity, than the brains of the rats from the other two groups. Thus, increased stimulation had resulted in increased brain growth.

ii Environmental deprivation

Goldman states that the strongest evidence to support the concept of environmental influence on brain development has come from the studies of selective stimulation or deprivation of a single sense (see note 25 above). The most striking results have been obtained by looking at the effects of deprivation on the visual system[30,31,32]. Almost all of these studies show that, with a decrease in visual stimulation, there is a depressive effect on visual function. Also, it was found that the early visual environment can modify the structure and function of connections in various regions of the visual system.

iii Environmental enrichment following brain injury

One of the first people to investigate this area was Schwartz.[33] He studied four groups of rats – those who received brain injury one day after birth and were then placed in either an enriched or normal environment, and rats without brain injury who were placed in either of the same two environments.

After 120 days, all the rats were tested. It was found that not only did the brain injured rats from the enriched environment perform better than the brain injured ones who had been in the normal environment, but they also did as well as the rats with intact brains who had been in the normal environment. In other words, increased stimulation in these rats after brain injury resulted in normal levels of performance.

This experiment was repeated[34,35,36] to see if the enriched conditions following brain injury would affect brain size and chemistry, as well as performance. Since Schwartz had only studied rats injured immediately after birth, the effects on older rats were also investigated. These studies showed that, even though brain injury had occurred, the increased stimulation did in fact produce larger brain weights and increased chemical activity, just as it had done with the normal rats. These same results were also evident in young adult rats – those over 100 days of age.

Thus, following brain injury, the amount of environmental stimulation provided plays a vital role in determining how much brain growth and recovery of function will occur.

iv Human studies

Obviously, most of the environmental studies we have reported cannot be carried out with human subjects, as they require exposing people to deliberate sensory deprivation, and in some instances involve removing the brain at the end of the testing period.

However, there have been tragic situations where humans have had to endure extreme sensory deprivation. Occasionally, children have been discovered after spending long periods confined to a tiny room, or even locked in a cupboard. In almost all of these cases, the children were found to have serious neurological deficits as a result of the environment they were forced to live in.

White[37,38], writing in 1966 and again in 1969, was able to study the effects of an enhanced environment on a group of normal infants. Working with institutionalized illegitimate children, he found that those placed in an environment enriched by increased visual and motor stimulation, achieved visual-motor skills, such as reaching out and grabbing, at a much faster rate than those exposed to a normal environment.

v Some possible explanations

Will and associates (see notes 35, 36 above) postulate that enriched experience may help to overcome the effects of brain injury in at least three ways:

1. It results in an increase in the number of connections and pathways in the brain, which may in part take over the functions of the destroyed or damaged tissue.
2. It may protect against the secondary loss of cells in regions away from the injured site-cells that through reorganization may be able to take over function. Their studies showed that the loss of these cells was somewhat smaller in the enriched group.
3. It may promote a compensatory increase in the vital brain chemicals which determine brain growth, since their studies also showed that the measure of these chemicals was larger in the enriched group.

Thus, through the various processes described in this chapter – reorganization of brain tissue, the use of redundant pathways, collateral sprouting, the response to increased environmental stimulation – and perhaps by other methods not yet understood, the enormous spare capacity that exists in the brain can be utilized.

It can now be said that the brain is in fact a dynamic organ, capable of a great deal of self repair.

CHAPTER SEVEN

Redirecting the Call

A T ONE time or another, most people have had some difficulty with their telephone service. Depending on what country you live in, the problem can range from being mildly annoying to totally frustrating. But, all things considered, the communications network that spans the globe is a marvellous achievement of modern technology. To be able to pick up a telephone, dial, and in a matter of seconds be talking to the other side of the world, is truly amazing.

When something goes wrong with the telephone, it serves as a reminder of how dependent we have become on this form of communication.

By looking at such a breakdown, and the response to it, we can get an idea of the sort of action needed when there is a 'breakdown' in the system that relays messages in the brain.

Suppose you are a business person in an office in Melbourne, and you want to telephone a client in New York. As your telephone is connected to the direct dialling system, such a process would be quite simple. Providing there were no breakdowns, you could be talking to your client within thirty seconds of picking up the telephone.

However, on this day, something is wrong with the direct line. As you are dialling, a recorded voice comes on to say that, due to a system malfunction, it is not possible to connect your call. Your next move would be to call the international operator to see if you can get through to New York. But the operator informs you that there is a complete shutdown of telecommunications between Australia and the USA.

You *must* get through, as there is a multi-million dollar contract hanging in the balance, so you ask the operator to find another way of making the call, regardless of how long it takes or how much it costs. Luckily, the operator rings back in a little while to say that she has found an alternate route to New York – via Sydney, Tokyo and Alaska.

It is more expensive and time consuming than the direct method, but you immediately give your approval for her to make the call this way. Fifteen minutes later, she rings you back with your New York client on the line.

What would have happened if our business person was not so determined, and he gave up after being told that the direct line to New York was out of order? Or if he struck an operator who could not be bothered investigating the different means of reaching New York, or who was new at the job and wasn't aware of the alternate routes available?

The telephone system would have been cursed for ever, and the talk would have been of the deal that got away.

Now, let's suppose that for some unknown reason, the direct communication link between Australia and the USA could never be restored. The only contact available would be through the route used by the business person – via Tokyo and Alaska. This alternate link would then be used a great deal, and with this frequent use, what was originally a cumbersome method would soon become very efficient.

Instead of having to discover an alternate route each time a call was made, as the first operator did, the response would become automatic. Since the exchanges in Tokyo and Alaska would suddenly have to handle all the Australia-USA calls, new operators would be put on to deal exclusively with these calls. With this continual use, the alternate route may eventually become so efficient that it would be almost as quick as the direct line.

This is exactly the same process that has to be established in an injured brain. The original connections have been destroyed and cannot be repaired, given that it is impossible to grow new brain cells.

But, as the scientific research described in the last two chapters has shown, there are many other 'operators' and new connections available, which, if they can be reached, possess the potential of accepting and redirecting the call.

The ultimate objective of such a process would be to make the new connections as efficient as possible, or even as good as the system which they replace.

Just as with the telephone call to New York, if such a system can be established its effectiveness depends largely on the persistence of the caller, the cooperation of the operator, the availability of new routes, and the number of times the newly established pathways are used.

The immediate problem is also the most overwhelming: how can we reach those potential alternate routes and put them into action?

Section III
The Importance of Normal Development

CHAPTER EIGHT

A Lesson from Nature

THE realization that the human brain is in fact a highly adaptable organ, with an enormous spare capacity, demands that the question of recovery of function following brain injury be looked at in a new light. It would seem that the spare capacity and plasticity of the brain is an integral part of its structure – possibly nature's compensation for the inability to grow new cells. If this is so, it could be said that following brain injury, there remains an enormous number of non-specific neurons that are apparently unaffected by the injury. These cells may possess the potential to become functioning neurons, and so take over from the destroyed cells.

It is important to note that even in the case of severe brain injury, where there has been no spontaneous recovery, this spare capacity still probably exists – since it appears to be an integral part of the brain. That this spare capacity has not been utilized may be due to at least two factors:

● The severity of the injury may have been so great that it prevented any spontaneous recovery from occurring.

● Treatment which may aid in the activation of this spare capacity may have been insufficient, inappropriate, or non-existent.

Given these two factors, the lack of any significant improvement does not automatically mean that the child is 'hopeless'. Even though spontaneous recovery has not occurred, it may still take place if an intensive therapy program is instituted. With such children, all avenues of treatment should be thoroughly investigated before the child's future prospects can be determined. When faced with the problem of restoring function after brain injury, the task at hand is to find a way of activating the reserve of non-specific brain cells and literally teaching them the functions of the destroyed cells which they have to replace.

How can these cells be reached? Given the present level of medical technology, they cannot be activated by drugs or surgery. Thus, the two major weapons of modern medicine are unable to achieve the desired result. Is it any wonder that for a long time such a process was thought to be impossible?

Again, we need to turn to recent scientific research for some answers – this time to work done concerning the recovery of function in rats following brain injury. The results of this work give an important insight into how the spare capacity of the brain can be utilized.

American scientists, Teitelbaum, Cheng and Rozin[1,2], published two interesting reports of their research. They studied the development of feeding in normal rats. To gain a better understanding of how this occurred, they created injuries to the feeding part of the brain, so they could observe any recovery of function that may take place.

As they watched the rats relearning how to feed, their curiosity was aroused. It seemed that all the rats were following the same sequence of recovery, with the speed of recovery being determined by how much injury was inflicted. Since the scientists were very familiar with the way feeding developed in normal rats, they were able to make another important observation. It appeared that the common sequence of recovery, followed by all rats after injury, resembled the sequential development of feeding that occurred in normal rats.

They then proposed that a parallel did exist, in fact, between the stages of recovery and normal development. To test this hypothesis, they closely studied two groups of rats. In one group, all of the rats were given exactly the same type of injury to the feeding part of the brain, with the rest of the brain left intact. Since it was observed that the brain injured rats passed through the developmental stages at a slower rate than normal, the second group consisted of normal rats whose development had been slowed down by a thyroid operation. If there was a parallel between stages of recovery and normal development, the two groups should develop in the same way, and at the same rate.

To the delight of the scientists, this in fact is what happened. The development of feeding in the two groups was remarkably parallel, thereby demonstrating that the recovery of feeding after brain injury followed the normal development sequence. This was a natural response, for there were no 'rat therapists' around to show the brain injured rats what to do. In explanation of their discovery, the scientists said that 'recovery recapitulates ontogeny'. Or, in other words, the process of recovery involved going back through normal development.

To make sure that their results were correct, the scientists repeated the study. This time, they slowed down the growth of the normal rats by starving them, rather than operating on the thyroid. Exactly the same results were achieved, once again confirming their original hypothesis.

There is evidence to suggest that this relationship between recovery from brain injury and normal development also exists in humans. Thomas E. Twitchell[3,4], a United States neurologist, studied the restoration of hand function following brain injury in adult humans. He observed that if they did regain the use of their hands, the process of recovery always followed much the same sequence – a sequence that was parallel to the development of hand function in normal infants. Twitchell made the observation that in a human system, 'adult recovery recapitulates infantile development'. This was the same conclusion as that made by the scientists working with the development of feeding in rats.

Teitelbaum[5] also made the comment, based on his own observations, that the recovery of voluntary hand control in humans, following frontal lobe damage, paralleled the development of such voluntary control in infancy. Ommaya[6], a United States neurosurgeon, has observed many severe head injury patients recovering from prolonged periods of unconsciousness. He has noticed that these patients appear to retrace, in their general behaviour and neurological pattern, their own growth and maturity. Ommaya describes this recovery as 'an often distorted and irregularly accelerated reproduction of normal development'.

The relationship between recovery and normal development can also be seen at a cellular level. Raisman[7] observed that the process of axon regeneration and collateral sprouting that occurs after injury to the brain, shows a distinct resemblance to the process of the 'wiring up' of the brain that occurs during normal development.

Therefore, it seems clear that there is an instinctive response that can occur in humans and animals following brain injury. In an effort to recover function, an attempt is sometimes made to go back through the stages of normal development – specifically through the stages that are appropriate to the level and type of injury sustained.

Moore[8], a United States anatomist, uses the story of the elderly father of a friend to illustrate this point very clearly. As a result of a severe stroke, this man became paralysed down one side, and he was sent home to live out his days as a bedridden cripple. But he refused to give up, and literally crawled out of bed each day on his hands and knees and went out into his garden. As well, he used this mode of transport to move around his house. This went on for the spring and summer, and after some time, he was able to stand up on his knees. Eventually, he was able to get up on his feet, and he began to cruise around the furniture. After some time, he was able to stand independently. Finally, he learnt to walk unaided. Thus, after several years, he had virtually rehabilitated himself and was able to function almost normally. According to Moore: 'Little did he know that he was 'instinctively' following the phylogenetic and ontogenetic growth and development patterns akin to those he had used subcortically when he was an infant, toddler, and young child.'

Is it possible that Nature has found a way of activating the vast reserve of non-specific brain cells that need to be utilized if recovery of function is going to occur? Is this why the instinctive response after brain injury seems to involve going back through normal development? Could it be that the process of normal development activates non-specific brain cells, and, if so, can this process be applied to the treatment of brain injury?

Normal development is something that most people take for granted, since most of the time it 'just happens', without the parents having to interfere. But there must be more to it than that. There has to be a reason why Nature goes back through development after the brain is injured.

If Nature tries to recapitulate normal development following brain injury, we need to try and understand why. We need to take a closer look at the process of normal development, and in particular, look at its relationship to the growth and development of the brain.

CHAPTER NINE

The Development and Organization of the Human Brain

IN NEARLY all cases, the growth that occurs in plants and animals is a result of an increase in the number of cells of that organism. However, the human brain is an exception to this rule, for the total number of neurons or nerve cells is developed before birth. Therefore, any growth that does occur after birth cannot be due to an increase in the cell number.

However, a considerable amount of brain growth does take place after birth. According to Stephen Rose[1], a British biologist, the brain of a newborn human weighs about 350 grams, compared with the adult weight of 1,300 to 1,500 grams. Most of this brain growth is completed by the tenth year of life, with the major growth occurring in the first couple of years. At six months, the brain is already 50 per cent of its eventual adult weight. At twelve months it is 60 per cent of this weight, 75 per cent at two-and-a-half years, 90 per cent at six years, and 95 per cent at ten years.

The brain's quadrupling in weight is partially due to the increase in the number of glial cells, a type of brain cell, which, unlike the neuron, is not involved in the transference of information in the brain. The weight increase also indicates a change in the neuronal network. The neurons grow in size, and become myelinated (myelin is a protective coating around the nerve fibres). As well, a vast network of blood vessels is established to supply vital nutrients to the brain. As the brain is 'wired up', an amazingly complex system of nervous connections is created in response to the sensory input coming into the brain, and to the motor reactions that are required. Thus the whole neuronal network increases dramatically in its size and complexity.

The human brain is remarkably immature at birth. Although all the cells that will eventually become functioning neurons are present, most of these are non-specific in the beginning. The cortex of the brain consists primarily of the Class II neurons, cells which at birth are largely unspecified and open to environmental influences, and which require stimulation for the development and maintenance of their function. Through the process of normal development, some of these cells become specific functioning neurons.

Thus, as a direct result of the sensory input and motor performance involved in normal development, neurons which were initially non-specific are activated, and an immature nervous system eventually becomes highly specialized and extremely complex.

This is the exact same process that has to be achieved if recovery of function is to occur following brain injury. A vast reserve of non-specific cells has to be stimulated into action and 'trained' to take over the functions of the destroyed cells. Drugs or surgery cannot activate non-specific neurons, but normal development can. This would appear to be the reason why Nature attempts to recapitulate normal development after brain injury, for it is a proven method of utilizing otherwise non-specific cells.

But, even in normal development, the growth of the brain is not an automatic process. As we have mentioned in the environment deprivation studies described in Chapter 6, when the brain is denied the appropriate stimulation and opportunity for expression, its development can be adversely affected. However, to a certain degree, development seems to happen despite the absence of proper environmental stimulation. Perhaps this is in part due to the function derived from the Class I neurons, the principal neurons that form the primary connections in the brain – since these neurons are largely unaffected by any variations in the environment.

The Class II neurons are those which will be affected by variations in the environment, since they are vulnerable to outside influence and are dependent on proper stimulation for their development. Seeing that these cells comprise the major part of the cortex, and since the cortex is responsible for the more sophisticated aspects of human development, the higher levels of brain function would be those more likely to be affected by inadequate or inappropriate stimulation. A child may still learn to walk despite extreme environmental deprivation, but he may have difficulty with the higher cortical functions, things such as reading, writing, and proper speech.

Thus it is important that, as a child develops, he adheres to some kind of step-by-step plan to ensure that his brain receives all the necessary stimulation and opportunity for expression that is essential for his brain to develop to its fullest potential. In fact, this is what usually happens. Even though all children are individual, and there are slight variations in the way that they progress, they all follow the same general plan of development – provided they are given the appropriate stimulation and opportunity. Normal development is not a random process that varies according to each child. On the contrary, it is organized in a highly structured way.

This structure is very rigid in the early stages of growth, but it becomes more flexible with time. The embryonic development of the central nervous system follows an exact timetable that is fixed and never changing, so much so that the stages of its growth can be pinpointed to the day. For instance, at nineteen days gestation, the neural tube – the forerunner to the brain – closes and begins its development; at day fifty-two, the optic nerve is formed from the eye to the brain; by day fifty-three, the cerebral hemispheres begin to develop.[2]

This embryonic growth occurs in such a way that each stage builds on the stages before, in a gradual sophistication of the overall structure. Correct growth depends on the integrity of the prior levels, and any malformation of the lower structures is likely to adversely affect subsequent growth.

It would be strange if, after following such a precise timetable of embryonic and foetal growth, this precision was disregarded after birth. As would be expected, it does in fact continue, especially in the early stages of post-natal development. Many experts in child development have observed this phenomenon. Jerome Kagan[3], Professor of Human Development at Harvard University, says:

The sturdiest knowledge we have about the development of infants is the exquisitely invariant order in which they master complex motor coordinations. Although there are slight differences in the ages at which these capabilities are attained, the sequence of events is rarely altered.

Jean Piaget[4,5], the famous French psychologist, refers to definite stages that are involved in the development of intelligence. He has described these stages in relation to the time at which they occur, and how they contribute to intellectual development. He considers these stages to be fixed, and that one has to pass through them, in correct order, so as to develop normal intelligence.

Penelope Leach[6], a British psychologist and author of several child development books, discusses the importance of the developmental stages of speech:

Language develops in infants at widely varying rates, and therefore at a range of ages, but it develops in an invariate sequence. The basic learning may, under optimal conditions, be compressed into two or three years, with only extensions of vocabulary, and the meanings of complex abstract thought still remaining to be learned. Or the basic learning may stretch over the whole of childhood. At either extreme, the sequence is the same.

Frank Caplan[7], director of the Princeton Center for Infancy and Early Childhood in the United States, sees development as being, to some extent, 'a natural process of unfolding, with the same sequence of stages occurring in all babies everywhere'.

This is not to say that all babies follow the same rigid pathway without variation. Each child is an individual with its own genetic make-up, and each is raised in his own unique environment with varying amounts of stimulation, opportunity and love. All these factors will have a direct bearing on development. But, for all these differences, the sequence of development is rarely altered.

As the brain matures, the functions of the child become more sophisticated and more numerous; such functions would not be possible with a less mature brain. Thus the level of function is determined by the amount of maturation that has occurred. According to Professor Kagan (see note 3 above): 'The developmental control of the universal motor pattern and certain cognitive processes in infants, are to a large extent controlled by maturation . . . we mean that biological factors limit the earliest appearances of certain functions; that the order of appearance, given the appropriate inducing environment, is controlled by the growth of the central nervous system. This does not mean that experience is irrelevant.'

Indeed it does not! To Professor Kagan's statement we wish to add that the proper and complete maturation and organization of the brain is dependent on the child being exposed to appropriate and adequate stimulation. The child also needs to be given sufficient opportunity for expression of motor functions. This stimulation and expression should be in accordance with the orderly, sequential stages of normal development. Thus, it works both ways – development is dependent on brain maturation, but brain maturation is also dependent on development.

Looking at a couple of examples of how this works in a normal situation will make this point clearer. Take, for instance, a toddler learning to walk. When one considers all that is involved in walking for the first time – the balance, strength, coordination and control – it's no wonder that it is not until around twelve months that the first steps are taken. Yet you never really have to teach a normal baby how to walk, for he is able to learn this by himself. This learning does not begin at the point where he starts pulling up on furniture and experimenting with being on two feet, nor does it happen when mum or dad 'walk' him around by supporting his upstretched arms. The foundations for the eventual achievement of walking are established as the baby learns to tummy crawl, roll, crawl on hands and knees, sit, and pull up on furniture and cruise along. All these skills help to develop and organize the mobility part of the brain, so that it will reach the level of maturity which enables the function of walking to occur.

If we look at normal development in this way, a baby doesn't crawl around on his tummy or hands and knees just to get from point A to point B. He also does this because it helps to ensure the proper development of his brain. This is obviously not a conscious decision on his behalf – he doesn't lie there and say to himself 'Well, today I'd better move around a little so as to fire a few more neurons into action'. Nature has already taken care of this – the everyday activities of the child are the means of developing the brain.

If the early developmental stages of movement weren't so important, they would have been discarded a long time ago and humans would get up to walk very soon after birth, just as do most other animals. However, most humans do not walk until at least twelve months, and this new function usually occurs after the lower movement stages have been perfected and used for several months.

Of course, there are exceptions. Some children learn to walk without passing through some of the lower stages, or they miss them altogether. However, an article in the *Australian Parents and Children* magazine[8] on the importance of crawling, says that often these children go back down on their hands and knees after they begin to walk: 'When they have been able to walk well for a few weeks, or even months, they will suddenly prefer to get about on all fours, crawling around as if they have never walked.'

Although some children can miss some or all of the lower movement stages and still be completely normal, this article goes on to say that problems can develop in some children who either do not crawl at all, or who only do it for a short period of time:

Their sense of balance or their ability to estimate distances is not as well developed as in other children. At five or six years of age they still have extreme difficulty in differentiating between right and left, catching a ball, or balancing on a chalk line.[8]

This clearly demonstrates that the lower stages of movement not only help the baby learn to walk – they have far greater implications concerning overall brain development. Such is the significance of crawling that the *Australian Parents and Children* article also says: 'There is also evidence of the importance of allowing babies to crawl a lot and for a long time, without constant encouragement to get up and walk properly'.

In fact, movement is the key that helps unlock the brain. Maria Montessori[9], the world renowned educator, expresses this belief very clearly:

Movement has great importance in mental development itself, provided that the action which occurs is connected with the mental activity going on. Watching a child makes it obvious that the development of his mind comes about through his movements. In the development of speech, for example, we see a growing power of understanding go side by side with an extended use of those muscles by which he forms sounds and words. Observations made on children the world over confirm that the child uses his movements to extend his understanding. Movement helps the development of the mind, and this finds expression in further movement and activity. It follows that we are dealing with a cycle, because mind and movement are parts of the same entity. The senses also take part, and the child who has less opportunity for sensorial activity remains at a low mental level.

As important as movement is, it has to be realized that all aspects of the normal development process are vitally important to ensure proper brain growth and maturation. Earlier in this chapter, we made reference to the fact that development is highly organized and structured, that all children follow the same general plan of development. We now need to look more closely at this general plan, so as to understand why children do the things they do as they grow.

CHAPTER TEN

How It's Meant to Happen

D IFFERENT developmental profiles have been designed over the years by experts in child development, and these have helped to give further insight into the way normal children grow. To effectively measure the level of function of a brain injured child, a developmental profile needs to compare that child to his normal peers. Just describing the child's disabilities, without any reference point to normal development, is simply stating the obvious. It gives no indication how the child is progressing as related to normal children, nor does it suggest that for improvement to occur, a pathway based on normal development needs to be followed.

The ideal profile should be designed so that it can be easily understood by parents and is able to record the child's progress. The most suitable tool we have found for assessing brain injured children is the Sandler-Brown Developmental Profile, devised by leading United States rehabilitation consultants, Art Sandler and Sandra Brown (see pages 66-67).

It has been divided into two major sections: the Afferent Sensory Pathways (afferent = going in), and the Efferent Motor Pathways (efferent = going out). In other words, it looks at the way information comes in and goes out of the brain. On the sensory side, the three major senses – vision, auditory and tactile – are detailed; on the motor side it describes the expressive functions of mobility, language, and manual competence or hand function.

In each of these areas of brain function, the developmental stages are listed, along with the approximate time when these stages normally appear. Since each child learns and grows at its own pace, the average rather than the exact times are given. All children develop differently, and there is a wide variation in the times when each skill is acquired – but there is a point where concern should be felt if the deviation is too far from normal.

The profile also lists the relationship between the level of brain

ENVIRONMEN[T]

	1	2	3	4	5	6
Brain level	MEDULLA AND SPINAL CORD	PONS	MIDBRAIN			(— — — —)
Age	BIRTH	BIRTH TO 3 MTHS	3 MTHS TO 6 MTHS	6 MTHS TO 9 MTHS	9 MTHS TO 12 MTHS	TO 18 MTHS
AFFERENT SENSORY PATHWAYS — Visual	Pupillary reflex	Biocular outline perception; Unified ocular movement	Seeing gross detail	Appreciation of fine detail	Initial binocularity	Identifying simple abstracts
Auditory	Startle reflex	Initial perception of sounds; Response to threatening sounds	Localization of sounds	Appreciation of environmental sounds	Understanding several single words	many words and phrases
Tactile	Babinski reflex	Vital sensation; Early proprioception; Awareness of temperature and discomfort	Localization of sensation	Gnostic sensation	Proprioceptive ability as related to balance and space; Awareness of 3rd dimension	Initial stereognosis
Sensory category	RECEPTION	PERCEPTION	APPRECIATION			
Sensory level	REFLEX	VITAL	MEANINGFUL			
EFFERENT MOTOR PATHWAYS — Mobility	Complete movement of all extremities	Initial crawling	Functional crawling culminating in cross pattern	Initial creeping culminating in cross pattern	Functional creeping culminating in cross pattern; Assume and maintain quadruped position; Pull to stand with fixed support	Cruising; Free standing; balance role
Language	Birth Cry	Vital sounds	Experimental use of sounds	Range of expressive and meaningful sounds	Word like sounds	meaningful words, however pronounced
Manual	Bilateral grasp reflex	Bilateral vital release	Initial prehensile grasp	Mature bilateral prehensile grasp	Unilateral cortical opposition	Bilateral cortical opposition; Unilateral cortical opposition; Initial bimanual function; tools

COPYRIGHT © SANDLER AND BROWN, 1981, SECOND EDITION

ENVIRONME[NT]

SANDLER-BROWN DEVELOPMENTAL PROFILE

------ CORTEX ------▶

BRAIN STAGE	AVERAGE TIME FRAME	VISION	AUDITORY	TACTILE	MOBILITY	LANGUAGE	MANUAL
12	6 YEARS TO PEER LEVEL	All visual abilities equal to or above peers, consistent with dominant hemisphere	All auditory abilities equal to or above peers, consistent with dominant hemisphere	All tactile abilities equal to or above peers, consistent with dominant hemisphere	All mobility functions equal to abilities equal to or above peers, consistent with dominant hemisphere	All language abilities equal to or above peers, consistent with dominant hemisphere	All manual and writing skills equal to or above peers, consistent with dominant hemisphere
11	5 YEARS TO 6 YEARS	Reading books	Sophisticated concept of time and space	Sophisticated stereognosis / Sophisticated proprioception	Hop, skip, jump, and other sophisticated skills	Sophisticated ability to express abstract thought	Writing many words spontaneously
10	4 YEARS TO 5 YEARS	Reading initial books	Conception of sophisticated abstract language	Concepts of solidity	Run and walk in complete cross pattern	Ability to participate in organized conversation / Proper articulation	Writing several words spontaneously
9	3 YEARS TO 4 YEARS	Reading sentences	Conception of grammatical and idiomatic language	Concepts of shape	Initial running in cross pattern	Structured sentences / Advancing vocabulary	Reproducing symbols and words
8	2 YEARS TO 3 YEARS	Reading phrases / Reading many words	Comprehension of worldly information leading to concept of time and space	Concepts of size	Initial walking in cross pattern	Initial sentences / Many phrases	Sophisticated bimanual skills
7	18 MTHS TO 24 MTHS	Reading several words / Identifying	Comprehension of basic directions	Concepts of texture	Walk and run with arms down without pattern	Initial phrases / Many new words	Bilateral and simultaneous cortical

CONCEPTION

UNIQUELY HUMAN PHYSICAL AND INTELLECTUAL SKILLS

maturity and the development of corresponding functions. Skills that develop at the time a certain level of the brain becomes operational are likely to be controlled by that level. For instance, the lower movement patterns of tummy crawling and crawling on hands and knees develop as the lower levels of the brain, primarily the midbrain, reach maturity. Thus, it would seem that the midbrain is responsible for these particular movement patterns.

Before we go any further, we have to clear up one area which is bound to cause confusion. On the Sandler-Brown profile, the movement a baby makes when he starts to move around on his tummy is described as 'crawling', and movement on hands and knees is called 'creeping'. However, most people think of a crawling child as one moving on hands and knees. Therefore, we need to establish a rule for this book regarding these terminologies. Even though the Sandler-Brown profile says otherwise, we will use 'crawling' to describe movement on hands and knees, and 'tummy crawling' to denote movement on the tummy. Therefore, as you read the profile, substitute tummy crawl for crawl, and crawling for creeping. We hope that this hasn't confused you even more!

As the profile progresses in an upward direction, it has been divided into four major levels, each one corresponding to a specific level of brain maturation.

Compared to most other animals, a newborn human is a helpless bundle. This is because the brain is at a very low level of maturity – it has yet to be 'wired up'. Although recent research has shown that a newborn has more ability than previously thought, in general, the brain is operating at a primitive reflex level. Most of its response to light, and sound and touch is reflexive, and most physical movement occurs without any real control.

These reflexes, as primitive as they may seem, are vitally important to the future development of the brain, for they form the foundation stones from which all function develops. The continual stimulation of these reflexes opens and develops the pathways in the brain. The environmental deprivation studies discussed in Chapter 6 suggest that if a baby is placed in an environment where these reflexes are not adequately stimulated, later development can be detrimentally affected.

For instance, if a newborn is placed in a completely dark room and left there for twelve months, in all likelihood the child will be blind or have very poor vision at the end of this time. The pupillary reflex – the constriction of the pupils in response to bright light – will not have been stimulated, and the visual part of the brain will have received insufficient input for it to function properly. Likewise, if a newborn is placed in a completely soundproof room and left there for twelve months, he will most probably be deaf after this time. The startle reflex – the reflexive response to a sudden loud noise – will not have been stimulated, and the higher auditory areas will receive no input, and thus the auditory part of the brain will be improperly developed.

Piaget[1] recognized the vital importance of this reflexive stage of development. According to him, a baby's functional level at birth consists of a small number of somewhat clumsy, unfinished, and isolated reflexes that are the foundation elements of all later intelligence. By documenting the development of his own three children, Piaget described and explained the emergence of problem-solving and thinking ability in the first two years of life – all of which he said originated from the seemingly random and inconsequential reflex actions at birth.

From birth to three months, the Pons level of the brain becomes completely functional. Development is also occurring in the higher brain levels during this time, but not yet to the point where these higher levels can begin to assert control. At this point, the baby begins to perceive his environment, but he is still operating at a rather primitive stage of maturation. Since the pathways are immature, the brain is more likely to receive input from stronger stimulants, rather than softer ones. Thus, the baby is more likely to respond to loud noises than to quiet ones, bright rather than soft lights, and unpleasant instead of pleasant stimulation.

At this stage, probably more than at any other level in development, the dependence of motor functions on proper sensory input is most obvious. The baby is beginning to perceive the environment, but cannot really comprehend the information that he is receiving. Since the more intense stimulants register in the brain first, the baby now has a reason to exhibit a motor reaction. In response to a sometimes scary and unpleasant world, the baby develops protective motor responses. He begins to use crying as a way of letting mum or dad know that the loud noises bother him, or that the safety pin which was accidentally stuck into him really did hurt. If he is in an uncomfortable position, or is too close to something that is unpleasant, his perception of this discomfort or threat gives him a reason to try and move away or change his body position. Since he is able to feel pain, he also has a reason to release a painful object from his grasp.

All of these motor responses are dependent on the baby being able to properly perceive the environment through his senses. If he could not feel any pain or discomfort, he would have no reason to cry or release an object from his grasp. If he could not see, feel or hear anything, there would be little or no incentive to begin to move. Thus, sensory input plays a major role in the development of motor functions.

At this point, the baby is really starting to appreciate the world around him. No longer is it just the bright, loud and unpleasant things that he is most responsive to, for now he sees things in detail, can locate and understand sounds and enjoys being touched and stroked.

Again, an appropriate motor response to sensory input can be observed. The three- to nine-month-old baby begins to establish purposeful motor patterns so that he can explore the world that is unfolding before his very eyes, his ears and his skin. He starts to move around so that he can investigate everything around him, he begins to communicate his needs in order to get what he wants, and he develops the ability to reach out and grab what he sees.

From nine months on, the cortex undergoes a period of amazing growth and maturity, and its continued development eventually results in the acquisition of the uniquely human functions of reading, writing, speaking and understanding language. It becomes the master of the central nervous system, the commander-in-chief of the lower parts of the brain. Since the development of the cortex is a complex procedure, it naturally takes time. There are many stages to go through before the optimum level is reached. As with the lower parts of the brain, the cortex follows an organized, hierarchical pattern of development, building on to the maturation that has already occurred.

Although the cortex is the major part of the brain, the lower levels play an essential role in its growth. They lay the foundations upon which the cortex builds – the cortex enlarges and sophisticates the development that has already taken place at the lower brain stages.

This has been an overview of development. We now need to look more closely at how each function develops.

Vision
Level 1 Pupillary reflex

If you shine a bright light into a newborn's eyes, the pupils will constrict. When the light is turned off, they will dilate back to their previous size. This is a reflex reaction that remains throughout life.

Level 2 Biocular outline perception

It is now realized that the visual abilities of a newborn are much greater than was previously thought. According to Frank Caplan[2]: 'Newborns see – they are visually sophisticated organisms'. Work such as that by Robert Fantz[3] has shown that within twelve hours of birth, babies can discriminate between a plain grey disc and an identical disc striped in black and white, if it is placed less than 23 cm (nine inches) from the bridge of the nose – and they prefer the striped disc to the plain one.

Penelope Leach[4,5], states: 'Babies can see, clearly and with discrimination, from the moment of birth'. But she points out that their visual abilities have long been underestimated simply because they are extremely short-sighted. In fact, research has shown that their functional vision is limited to objects that are less than 20-23 cms (eight to nine inches) from the bridge of the nose. Research by Janet Atkinson and her colleagues[6] has shown that this short range of vision is not because babies cannot adjust their focusing to varying distances, as was first thought, but that they usually do not. They have the ability, but in the beginning they cannot use it accurately and consistently, for it takes time to develop this control. At nine days, 80 per cent of the babies they studied could focus accurately at two-and-a-half feet, but only 50 per cent did so, and only 20 per cent ever focused at five feet. By three months, 80 per cent could focus at five feet, and 75 per cent did so consistently.*

While recognizing that a newborn possesses close range visual ability, the Sandler-Brown profile measures *functional* vision. Given that most of the world is further than 23 cm from a baby's eyes, a newborn's visual skills are not yet functional. Thus, the profile measures the ability of a baby to react visually to objects

* [One foot = 30.5 centimetres.]

other than those at very close range. From birth to three months, biocular outline perception develops. The infant will follow objects that move across his field of vision – initially just those at close range, but later, those further away. Even if the objects he sees are blurry, he will still track them.

Level 3   Unified ocular movement, seeing gross detail

As a baby begins to follow objects at a distance, the eyes may not always work together. According to Caplan: 'Beyond that range (20-23 cms), he probably has only a hazy image and his eyes may wander independently, or flare outward for a while'. But, between three and six months, the eyes begin to work in proper coordination at any distance.

At this time, his range of vision increases dramatically – he begins to focus on and recognize objects that are further and further away. He not only recognizes faces, but displays established preferences for certain people, especially his mother. In the early stages of vision, a baby is most responsive to the human face, but by six months he will recognize other important things in his life, such as the breast or bottle. He displays reasonable hand-eye coordination, and is quite sociable with lots of smiles and laughter.

Level 4   Appreciation of fine detail

From six to nine months, the infant develops purposeful and functional vision. He can recognize more people, his favourite toys, his dummy, food, etc. He also develops the ability to see very small objects, and may become fascinated with such things as tiny crumbs on his plate.

Level 5-6   Initial binocularity, complete convergence of vision

There is no need to worry if a six-month-old's eyes don't look exactly straight as he focuses on an object. This precise control of the eyes takes time to develop, and is not completely mastered until the child is twelve to eighteen months old. This control gives the child convergence of vision – the eyes work exactly in unison, resulting in depth perception.

Level 6-7   Identifying simple abstracts, identifying complex symbols, reading several words

By eighteen to twenty-four months, a child has the neurological ability to identify simple pictures, letters, numbers, and several words. Yes – surprising as it may seem, children this young do have the ability to learn to read.

How this can be taught to children of this age is the subject of Chapter 23.

Level 8-12 The sophistication of reading
If reading is taught at an early age, a child should be able to read simple books by the time he is six. As this skill develops, he goes through the stages described in levels 8-12.

Auditory
Level 1 Startle reflex

As with the pupillary reflex, there is an auditory response present at birth that continues through life – the startle reflex. This is a reflexive response to a sudden loud noise, and is usually a jumping reaction.

Level 2 Initial perception of sounds, response to threatening sounds
Babies seem to respond to two kinds of sounds in the first months of life. They are soothed by rhythmical sounds such as gentle music, humming and soft tapping and hearing a recording of the mother's heartbeat and placental sounds can soothe crying babies to sleep. But if the baby is already content, he initially responds more to louder sounds than to softer ones.

A loud sound will often cause a baby to startle and cry – a normal protective response.

Level 3 Localization of sounds
By three to six months, a baby not only hears most sounds, but is now able to locate the direction from which they are coming and turn his head and body towards the source.

Level 4 Appreciation of environmental sounds
By six to nine months, the infant's hearing is very acute, and he responds to most sounds around him. He also understands the meaning of familiar sounds. For instance, if he hears the sound of

running water coming from the bathroom, he associates this with bath time.

Level 5 Understanding several single words
As the auditory pathway becomes more sophisticated, the nine- to twelve-month-old begins to understand his first words. These are the words that he hears most often – his name, mummy, daddy and 'no' – a word he has been hearing a lot of since his discovery of all the wonderful things which babies aren't supposed to touch.

Level 6 Understanding many words and phrases
By eighteen months, the infant is understanding a lot of what is being said to him. He can comprehend many different words, and can understand short phrases. At this point he is able to follow simple directions – if he wants to!

Level 7-12 The sophistication of understanding
By the time children reach the age of six, they have an excellent understanding of human speech. On the way to this level, they pass through the stages described in levels 7 to 12.

Tactile
Level 1 Babinski reflex

There are different skin reflexes present at birth, with the Babinski reflex being the one used on the profile. When the sole of a newborn's foot is stroked, the toes turn out and the big toe shoots up in the air. This is a reflex response, and is not indicative of the sensation of touch.

Level 2 Vital sensation, early proprioception, awareness of temperature and discomfort
The newborn is very responsive to skin contact, and especially to being held – this is usually very soothing. But the sensations that produce the first appropriate motor responses are the stronger, more unpleasant ones. The baby is bound to cry if he is accidentally pricked with a pin, or if the bath water is too hot. Also, he begins to feel the movements that occur in his limbs, and he starts to develop initial body awareness or proprioception.

Level 3 Localization of sensation
From three to six months, the sense of touch becomes more acute. The infant will withdraw his arm or leg if this part of his body receives an unpleasant stimulus, as he is now able to localize where the sensation is being applied.

Level 4 Gnostic sensation, proprioceptive ability as related to balance and space
The infant at six to nine months can now appreciate light touch (gnostic sensation), and he becomes ticklish. His proprioceptive or balance sense develops to the point where he can sit independently, and balance on all fours.

Level 5 Awareness of third dimension
As the sense of touch develops further, the nine- to twelve-month-old discovers that objects have a third dimension – depth. As he intently explores a button on his mother's dress with his fingers, he is discovering that touch is another way of learning about the world around him.

Level 6-7 Initial stereognosis, concepts of texture
From this point, the infant begins to develop the sense of stereognosis, the ability to identify objects by feeling. This begins with the differentiation between textures, and the infant becomes fascinated with the different surfaces and feelings that he comes across.

Level 8-12 The sophistication of stereognosis
With time, the stereognostic ability of a child becomes highly developed. For instance, a five- or six-year-old can put his hand into a bag of toys, and pull out his favourite, without having to look at it. A blind person is a good example of how refined stereognosis can become, as much of the information about his environment comes through his sense of touch.

Mobility
Level 1 Complete movement of all extremities

A newborn's limbs can be moved through a full range of movement without any abnormal muscle tone being felt. During the uncontrolled reflexive movement that occurs, the newborn's limbs should move freely. There is virtually no control of movement at this point, although a baby can turn his head to one side to avoid smothering when on his tummy.

Level 2 Initial tummy crawling

During the first three months, although the baby's movements are uncontrolled, he is learning about his body and what is involved with movement. If he spends a lot of time on his tummy on the floor, by three months initial rolling movements may have begun, and he will be starting to work out what is required to move forward.

Level 3 Functional (tummy) crawling culminating in cross pattern

The first attempts at forward movement are unrefined, and progress can be measured in centimetres. The initial movements may be in a circle or even backwards, but eventually he will go in the right direction. Different patterns of movement may be used, but most infants end up moving in cross pattern, as this is the most efficient way of tummy crawling. This involves using opposite sides of the body together, so that he pulls with the right arm while pushing with the left leg, and vice versa.

Level 4 Assume and maintain quadruped position, initial creeping (crawling)

From six to nine months, as the infant moves around on his tummy, he begins the first stages of the movement that will soon supersede his present mode of transport. He starts to try and get himself up on his hands and knees, although it doesn't look like this initially. He may lift his bottom in the air and bring his knees up underneath, or he may push up on his arms and lift his chest off the ground. Eventually, he puts it all together and supports himself on all fours in the quadruped position. As he starts to feel confident, he will begin rocking backwards and forwards, and he will soon try to take a few tiny steps forward.

Level 5 Pull to stand with fixed support, functional creeping (crawling) culminating in cross pattern

For the nine- to twelve-month infant, crawling on hands and knees is a very difficult skill to acquire, as strength, balance and coordi-

nation are all involved. As with tummy crawling, different movement patterns may be tried, usually culminating in cross pattern.
As crawling becomes very efficient, the first attempts at standing
occur as the infant pulls up to stand against furniture or anything
that offers suitable support.

Level 6 Cruising, free standing, walk with arms in primitive balance role

As more and more time is spent upright, balance and control in this
position improves to the point where cruising begins – sideways
walking around furniture and, with more practice, along a wall.
Then, free standing develops as the infant lets go of the furniture or
wall for brief periods. Eventually, the first teetering walking steps
are taken.

Level 7-12 The sophistication of walking

Soon, the child is walking everywhere. His coordination and balance
rapidly develop, and he begins running. By the time he is six, all his
movements will be very fluent and controlled.

Language
Level 1 Birth cry

Providing there are no complications, it is normal for the newborn
to cry or whimper. This cry is reflexive, and is not significant in
terms of communication.

Level 2 Vital sounds

In the beginning, the only language ability a baby has is crying. It
may seem strange to describe crying as being a language, but
according to Penelope Leach[4], crying forms a language in the sense
that with all infants hunger cries have one typical pattern, pain cries
another, and so on. Most mothers learn to interpret their baby's
cries fairly early, thus establishing a primitive form of communication.

Level 3 Experimental use of sounds

Even before three months, a baby will start to experiment with
sounds other than crying. But from three months on, this ability
really blossoms – he spends a lot of his waking time babbling, and

his repertoire of sounds gradually increases. While infants from three to six months recognize and respond to the social intent behind talking, there is no direct imitation of adult speech. During the course of babbling, word-like sounds may come out and the adult listener may think that the baby is trying to say a word, but this is more by accident than intention.

Level 4 Range of expressive and meaningful sounds
As a result of the practice gained during babbling, by six months the infant has developed a good range of sounds. At this point, he will often carry out long babbling 'conversations' with his mother. By seven months, the babble includes two-syllable 'words', an advance on the more simple sounds made earlier. By the eighth to ninth month, this has progressed to the point where his conversations are not just repetitions of the same sounds, but can include phrases of four or more syllables, with very definite changes of emphasis and shifts of phrasing.

Level 5 Word-like sounds
From nine to twelve months, the range of sounds is so large, and the inflections so marked and varied, that it seems as if the infant is talking fluently, only in 'another' language. In fact, his first 'words' are part of this 'foreign' language – he may not be quite able to say 'drink', the best he can do is 'doo-doo'. The only time he ever makes this sound is when he is thirsty, so his parents quickly realize that this is his word-like sound for drink, and in this way, this sound functions as the real word. He will most probably develop several other word-like sounds before the real words come out.

Level 6 Several spontaneous, meaningful words, however pronounced
As long as his attempts at speech are appropriately recognized and rewarded, the infant will continue to use them. With this repetition, the sounds will become more and more like the actual words, until they are clearly recognizable as the real word. At this point, it is vital not to continually correct his attempts at words, as this may frustrate and discourage him.

Level 7-12 The sophistication of speech
From eighteen months on, the child's speech advances rapidly – by

two years he is beginning to put words together, by three he is starting to use short sentences. His articulation continually improves, as does the content and maturity of his speech.

Manual
Level 1 Bilateral grasp reflex

If you put your finger into the palm of a newborn baby, he will instantly grasp it very tightly – a response known as the 'grasp reflex'. This is a reflex, and is not a sign of strength or advanced hand function.

Level 2 Bilateral vital release
A couple of weeks after birth, a baby seems to have lost his hand strength, for no longer will he always grab tightly at something placed in his palm. This is not a backward sign. Initially he grasped and kept his grip simply because he didn't know how to let go; now he has developed vital release – the ability to let go – a necessary function in case he grabs something painful.

Level 3 Initial prehensile grasp
Recent research, to be discussed in the next chapter, suggests that in the first weeks of life babies have good control over reaching out, but that this skill deserts them, only to return several months later. By three months, a baby will swipe at any object, but without much control.

Over the next couple of months this control improves with practice, and hand-eye coordination gradually develops.

Level 4 Mature prehensile grasp
By six months, the infant will reach out well, and will delight in grabbing anything he can get to. At this point, he prefers a two-handed approach, but this gradually improves to the stage where he will reach with just one hand, without necessarily showing a preference for either hand.

Objects are grasped with the whole hand, rather than just between the thumb and forefinger.

Level 5 Unilateral/bilateral cortical opposition
From nine months on, an infant begins to use a pincer grasp, or

'cortical opposition', whereby he uses the thumb and forefinger to pick up small objects. As simple as it may seem, this is an important step along the way to to acquiring manual dexterity.

Level 6 *Initial bimanual function, primitive use of tools*
The twelve-month-old is starting to discover just how useful his hands are. He soon realizes that he can use them together, and his bimanual coordination progressively gets better. He also discovers the joy of trying to feed himself with a spoon, and once he realizes he can do this he will be very reluctant to let mummy take over – even though more food may end up on the floor than in his mouth.

Level 7-12 *The sophistication of hand function*
Manual dexterity progresses rapidly from eighteen months on. The infant begins more involved coordination activities, first by learning how to reach out simultaneously with both hands and pick up two objects using the pincer grasp on each hand, and then by using two hands together in bimanual skills. Soon, no jar lid or bottle cap will be too difficult, and he will begin meaningful and quite complex construction. By the time he is six, he should be able to write several words, as well as being able to draw and copy.

In the previous chapter, we mentioned the importance of the development of movement in relation to the overall growth and organization of the brain. By looking at the profile, it is possible to see the corresponding development related to each movement stage.

For instance, take the example of tummy crawling and the development of control over the hands, the eyes and body awareness. The arm movement involved in crawling is very similar to the action involved in reaching out; therefore, tummy crawling helps develop and reinforce the ability to reach out. Moving on the tummy creates friction between the body and the floor, thereby increasing tactility and stimulating body awareness. A baby learns to move his head from side to side when crawling on his tummy, and he also has to move his eyes in a horizontal arc as his head moves – this is the same type of eye movement used when following an object.

Thus, as the baby practises tummy crawling, he is reinforcing and enhancing development in other areas, so it is not just coincidence that these other functions develop and are refined at around the same time. These abilities can be acquired without the baby learning to tummy crawl, as evidenced by children who skip this movement stage and still develop normally, but they are firmly established by the process of tummy crawling.

The same type of relationship can be seen when the infant learns to crawl on hands and knees. He has to deal with balance and body position, since he is only supported by his hands and knees. This provides a great deal of stimulation to the proprioception sense part of the brain – a look at the profile shows that proprioreception develops at the same time as crawling. Of course, it also works the other way around – his advancing proprioception helps his crawling.

Once he is on his hands and knees, the vision part of his brain has to deal with depth perception. It has to determine how far he is off the ground, how far away his hand is, and how far he should move forward. It is not just coincidence that the brain function that enables the perception of depth – convergence of vision – develops at the same time as the infant gets up on his hands and knees. Convergence can develop quite normally in children who do not crawl, but its development is more assured in children who do.

Thus, it can be seen just how beautifully Nature has arranged everything. Normal development is not a random process, but rather an intricately designed system that helps to ensure the proper development of the brain. At each level, the different areas of development reinforce each other, and the combined effect of all the component parts lay the foundation for the next stage.

Important as each part is, the brain is highly adaptable, and it is possible for normal development to occur even if stages are missed for one reason or another. But, knowing how valuable and closely related each level is, and that problems can develop if stages are missed, everything should be done to make sure that children both normal and brain injured, follow the normal sequence of events.

Going through all the stages of normal development doesn't ensure a normal child, but it certainly helps.

CHAPTER ELEVEN

A Baby's Neurological Workshop

GIVEN that each child is an individual, and that each grows up in a different environment, how best to ensure that normal development does occur? Does one take a laissez-faire attitude and leave it mostly up to the child, or should a more active role be played by the parent?

As we see it, it is up to the parents to provide the best possible environment for their child, so as to help him develop to his fullest potential. For, if they don't, who will?

It sometimes has been said that parents who give their children lots of early stimulation are simply trying to create geniuses, or are taking them beyond their natural potential. For instance, Arnold Gessell[1], a renowned United States child development expert, says: 'So far as we know, enriching the child's environment and providing him with the fullest opportunities possible permits him to express himself at his very best, but it does not make him "better" or smarter or speedier than he was born to be'. But, how do we know just what a child was 'born to be'? This cannot be known beforehand, so every attempt should be made to ensure that he reaches his fullest potential. There is a risk that if a child's environment is not enriched, he might not reach this potential.

It appears that the early months are the ideal time to begin stimulating a baby. In referring to the previously unrecognized capacities of an infant, Jaroslav Koch[2], a Czechoslovakian psychologist, states: '. . . this rich potential for development exists in a baby for only a given period, and the optimum stage for its awakening is in early infancy. If the appropriate stimuli are lacking in early infancy then the potential for developing certain skills, abilities and characteristics gradually disappears'. Koch also adds that 'the objective of education should not be to accelerate development, but to fully utilize all your baby's potential from his earliest age'.

How does a parent learn to do such an important job? Can one enroll in a 'How to be a good parent' class at the local education centre? There are usually no such classes, which means that parents are not adequately taught how to best assist their child's development. Instead, most simply learn as they go, especially with the first child. They would dearly love someone to give them some sound advice – hence the abundance of child development books on the market.

Parenthood is so important, and yet parents are usually unprepared for what is required of them. The more knowledge they have of normal development, the easier and more enjoyable their task will be. Such knowledge would also be of great assistance to parents of brain injured children, since the principles of normal development are vital to the treatment of these children. Without this understanding, some of the advice given in this book may seem inappropriate. For instance, if through some peculiar circumstance, we had only a brief moment to advise the parents of a brain injured baby on the simplest and most effective single thing they could do for their child, all we would say is: 'Put him on the floor!'

Initially, such advice sounds a little strange. But with an understanding of normal development, it becomes quite logical. Of course, there are many other pieces of advice we would like to give, but given the situation where only one thing could be said, 'put him on the floor' is what it would be.

But, why the floor? Well, for a normal baby, the floor is where everything happens, especially in the first twelve months. It is his neurological workshop, the place where the brain learns about its body and about movement. It is where a great deal of brain development occurs.

Being on the floor means that a child is on the floor for significant periods of time during the day, most of this time lying on his tummy rather than his back. Lots of colourful, noisy toys should be put around the child, to make it as interesting and stimulating as possible, and to encourage attempts at movement.

As mentioned earlier, a newborn baby is a mass of reflexes. If you watch a four-week-old baby lying on his tummy, a lot of uncontrolled movement of the limbs, especially of the legs, will be observed. Although these movements seem to be without purpose, they are actually very important for the future development of sophisticated movement. After many weeks of the baby being on the floor, something interesting begins to happen – by accident rather than design.

As he is lying there with his arms and legs moving around quite randomly, just by chance his arm and leg may coordinate. As a result, his body may roll slightly, or move forward a fraction. If this occurred only once or twice, little useful information about movement would reach the brain. But if the child spends a lot of time on the floor, such accidental movements would happen repeatedly, and the brain will start to learn what is involved in achieving purposeful movement, eventually mastering all that is required to move forward.

You can see this process happening as you watch a baby experiment with different movements as he lies on the floor and struggles to move. The more often a baby is on the floor, the more he will experiment with reflexive movement and learn how to control it. It's quite simple – practice makes perfect.

Most babies, if placed on the floor from the beginning, enjoy being there. In fact, many parents have said that these children don't like being held for too long, as they want to get back down to where everything is happening. In the early weeks, a baby placed on his tummy on the floor may begin to cry after a while, since he is not yet used to being there, as well as the fact that he cannot yet lift his head up and look around. Therefore, in the beginning it is best to put him down for frequent short sessions rather than for one or two long ones. Besides, there are lots of other good things to be done with baby apart from just putting him on the floor.

The increased knowledge about the abilities that newborn humans possess serves to further strengthen the case for early stimulation. Of particular interest is the work of Thomas Bower[3], a psychologist at Edinburgh University. One of the things that he has demonstrated is that newborn infants show an extraordinary capacity for imitating adult behaviour. For instance, he has photographic proof of six-day-old babies imitating their mother poking out her tongue. Bower sees this ability as the most remarkable example of the competence of the newborn's perceptual system. He states: 'Consider what is involved in imitating someone sticking out their tongue. The infant must identify the thing he sees in the adult's mouth as being a tongue. He must realize that the thing he cannot see but can feel in his mouth is also a tongue, the homologue of the thing he sees. He must then execute fairly complex muscular movements in order to imitate what he sees.' Quite an achievement for a six-day-old baby!

But something strange happens to this seemingly precocious ability. According to Bower: 'In spite of the fact that the ability manifests itself so early in life, it soon seems to fade away, re-appearing only toward the end of the child's first year.'

Bower also observed other examples of this peculiar situation where skills existed much earlier than expected, only to disappear and then re-emerge at a later time. He closely studied the acqui-sition of hand function in infants[4,5]. As with their ability to imitate, he observed a surprising degree of reaching ability in newborn infants. He found that if a fourteen-day-old infant is fully awake, and supported in a semi-upright position so that the head and arms are free to move, he will reach out and grab visually presented objects. As well, infants of this age show a surprising amount of control, as their reaching had a success rate of about 40 per cent, with more than half their misses landing a hair-breadth away from the target object. Bower also observed that infants lying on their backs were less successful at reaching out and grabbing.

This reaching ability in very young infants has also been noted by other researchers. Butterworth[6], an English psychologist, said, after observing infants in a laboratory situation,

. . . there is little doubt that infants in the first few weeks of life can reach towards and sometimes grasp objects on which they fixate visually.

Another researcher, Trevarthen[7], has also observed this ability.

Since these observations obviously challenge the accepted notions of the functions of young infants, there is a great deal of controversy amongst child development experts as to whether this skill in fact does exist at such an early age. In critical studies, Dod-well, Muir and Di Franco[8,9] state they found no evidence to support the concept of early reaching in infants. However, Bower, and his associates Dunkeld and Wishart[10], defended their earlier findings by claiming that the experimental techniques used by Dodwell and his colleagues were flawed. Dodwell[11] then defended his techni-ques, saying that the initial instructions given by Bower, and then followed by Dodwell, were too vague. So, the controversy contin-ues!

Bower (see notes 3, 4, 5 above) also observed that just as the infant's ability to imitate disappeared, so too did his attempts at reaching out and grabbing. The appearance, disappearance, and subsequent reappearance of these skills intrigued Bower, so he set about studying this phenomenon. He wanted to find out why the earliest phase of gaining an ability – which he referred to as 'Phase 1' – came to an end, and to see if there was any relationship between Phase 1 and when the ability returned – 'Phase 2'.

He concentrated his study on the function of reaching out and grabbing. He gave infants intensive practice at this skill during Phase 1, which in this case was the first four weeks of life. Having done this, he then observed that in some of the cases, the Phase 2 stage appeared earlier than normal. In other words, if appropriate and adequate stimulation was given when the skill was first apparent soon after birth, it did not take as long to become firmly established as a permanent ability.

Even more significant was the observation that some of the infants did not lose the Phase 1 ability – being given the opportunity to reach for objects right from birth meant there was no decline in their reaching ability. The skill was established at Phase 1, thereby giving the infant an important exploratory function at an early age.

Bower believes that babies are born with much more ability than they are given credit for, and that such behaviour is seldom seen only because we do not expect it, and therefore do not facilitate it. His explanation of why infants lose early visual and motor abilities, only to regain them later, is that the opportunity is not given during Phase 1 to practise and reinforce these skills; hence they are lost, only to be relearned during Phase 2.

Despite the apparent reversals and repetitions, Bower still considers normal development to be a continuous, cumulative process, with appropriate stimulation and opportunity reinforcing the current level of development and leading to the next stage of skill acquisition.

So, what are the implications of this recent infant behaviour research? First and foremost, it shows that for too long, a newborn baby's abilities have been under-estimated. For instance, it has been assumed for a long time that babies do not see very much, but as we reported in an earlier chapter, it now seems that this is because we haven't realized how short-sighted they are. And we had thought that babies weren't able to reach out, but this may be because we have never given them the chance to do this. As

Bower's work demonstrates, such under-estimations have possibly made normal development that little bit more difficult and somewhat slower.

Most babies spend little time lying awake on their tummy in their first weeks and months. But this is the position from which functional movement, such as crawling and creeping, develops. Therefore, it would be a distinct advantage if they were given plenty of opportunity to feel and experiment with movement in this position.

Thus, we need to reassess how we look at the role of parents in child development. They are the ones responsible for raising the child, therefore they should be properly equipped for the tremendous task they are undertaking. The best tool they can be given comes in the form of education, especially about the importance of the early development stages. As well, they need to understand and appreciate the abilities of an infant so that they can best enhance the enormous potential that is lying there, waiting to be given the opportunity to blossom.

But, all the stimulation and opportunity provided has to be at the appropriate level. There is no point in teaching a two-month-old baby about nuclear physics – although this may sound ridiculous, Penelope Leach[12] points out that the way we provide visual stimulation for a baby may be similarly inappropriate:

We know, for example, that infants cannot see detail across the width of even the smallest room. We know too, that they choose to give their attention to what they have not seen before. So it seems a pity to waste nursery mobiles, pictures, brilliant wallpapers, and all the other accoutrements of a really interesting room on a baby who will not see the interesting features, but will probably see just enough to get bored with it all before his distance accommodation catches up. It would seem that such a room, organized when the infant was around four to six months, would give infinitely greater pleasure.

We know that babies like pictures of things; that they actually choose to give them their attention. Yet many a mother would feel ridiculous to sit a two-month baby on her lap and show him a big, bold picture book.

We know that infants focus best on objects between eight and 15 inches away from them, yet we seldom make use of this knowledge. Interesting things hung from the hood of the pram, for example, are usually too high for close inspection; mothers may even be afraid that putting them closer will make the baby squint. Even grandmothers, desperate for attention, are more likely to get him to smile if they will put their faces up to the baby's own.

Thus, the better the process of normal development is understood, and the infant's abilities recognized, the more enjoyable and rewarding parenthood will become – and the better will be the child's chances of developing his full potential. This applies as much to children who are brain injured as it does to those who are normal.

Section IV
How the Brain Can Be Treated

CHAPTER TWELVE
You Have To Walk Before You Can Run

'YOU HAVE to walk before you can run!' So say many parents, as they watch their over-anxious toddlers trying to move faster than their tiny legs and still developing brain enable them. Usually the child doesn't heed the warning as he is so intent on getting where he wants to go. As a result, he encounters many tumbles along the way.

Even so, the advice is wise. The child is being told exactly what was said in the last section – that human development is meant to occur in an orderly fashion, and it's best not to rush things or do them out of sequence. The child will learn to run once his coordination and balance have been developed to the required level by walking and going through the lower movement stages. Such advice is freely given to normal children, but often seems to be forgotten when dealing with those children who are brain injured. And yet, if their condition is to improve, many of the principles of normal development need to be incorporated into their treatment programs.

In the first place, these principles tell us that we have to recognize and understand the orderly and sequential pattern of normal development. So, when confronted with the task of restoring or developing a particular function lost through brain injury, one of the first questions that needs to be asked is: 'How does this function develop in normal children?' The stages required to develop that function initially are the means most likely to be the most efficient and effective in achieving that particular skill. Adopting such an approach almost invariably involves going back through the lower stages of development that a normal child experiences as this function is attained.

Moore[1] states that this concept needs to be applied to enable the lower or redundant levels of the brain to take over the function of the damaged higher areas. She states: 'However, these older CNS (Central Nervous System) systems cannot be "reawakened" by utilizing techniques that are applicable for rehabilitating the neo-systems (higher brain levels), i.e. the use of therapeutic measures that require a degree of conscious effort such as walking, dressing, eating, speaking, etc. Rather, these older systems need to be tapped and reinforced by having the patient use them in a manner in which they once functioned.'

Jean Ayers[2], a psychologist in the U.S.A., says much the same thing:

The course of therapy follows a similar progression (to normal development). Enhancing maturation at the lower, less complex levels of environmental-response function enables a child to become more competent at the higher, more complex areas.

The article from *Australian Parents and Children* magazine, mentioned in Chapter 9, concerning children who can develop problems if they miss the crawling stage also makes reference to the need to utilize normal developmental stages in therapy. It says:

These children must make up at this age for what they missed out on by not crawling in their first year of life, with the help of a therapist.

Answering the question 'How does this function develop in normal children?' requires looking at what stages a child goes through to achieve that particular skill.

Once the component parts have been established, methods have to be found by which these can be replicated – so that the brain injured child can be 'taken back' through these developmental stages.

To illustrate how this can be done, we would like to look at the case of 'Mary', a composite of many patients we have seen. This will provide only a broad outline of how these developmental principles can be put into practice, as each child has a unique set of problems, and responds in his own way to a given treatment technique.

Mary is three years old. She suffered a severe injury to her brain as the result of her mother's 'problem' pregnancy and a very difficult and traumatic delivery. Mary's brain injury is extremely severe, and it has resulted in almost total devastation in all areas. In fact, there is almost nothing she can do – she is blind, deaf, insensate, and has no motor function. To demonstrate how they can be treated, each of her functions needs to be looked at individually.

Vision

Mary has been diagnosed as 'cortically blind'. This means that there is nothing directly wrong with her eyes – she is blind because of damage to the visual cortex, the part of the brain that controls vision. It may sound strange that an attempt can be made to restore vision in a blind child, but if the blindness is due to injury to the brain rather than the eye, there is a possibility that visual function can be achieved.

Although Mary cannot see, her pupils still respond to light. Her reflex action is not normal, as the pupils only react to a very strong light, and even then the response is slow and incomplete. But, there *is* a response, and that gives something to build on. If we measured Mary on the Sandler-Brown profile, she would be at level one in vision.

Since Mary has no visual function other than the pupillary reflex, the treatment program would have to start right from the beginning. Luckily, it is easy to stimulate the pupillary reflex, as all that is needed is a bright light. In Mary's case, the light would have to be strong enough to make the pupils constrict, seeing that her reaction is slower than normal. The light has to be shone into her eyes for one second, this being long enough to cause the pupils to constrict. The light should then be switched off for five seconds, to give the pupils time to dilate in the dark. (This should be done in a dark area.) The light needs to be turned on and off in this manner for 20 times in each vision session, with the session then being repeated 20 to 30 times each day. Hopefully, as a result of all this stimulation, Mary's pupillary response to light will improve, a possible indication that the visual pathway is beginning to develop.

In accordance with how vision develops in normal children, the next level of Mary's vision that has to be developed is the ability to follow moving objects, and the capacity to see gross detail. This would initially be at close range, since in the beginning a baby's range of vision is limited to objects within 20–23 cms from the bridge of the nose. It would appear logical that as the first stages of Mary's vision developed, the same limitations of visual range would apply. Therefore, the stimulation provided to encourage following and detail vision would need to be given close to her eyes. As well, since research has shown that babies are most responsive to human faces, these should feature strongly in the toys and pictures used for stimulation.

In both the following and detail exercises, the intensity of the objects being used has to be increased in some way, as her vision at this point is still extremely limited. Somehow, she has to be shown objects that she almost can't help but see. Several very simple but effective techniques have been developed for this purpose. For instance, faces and pictures painted on white cardboard in fluorescent paint, and then put under ultra-violet light, are wonderful for highlighting and bringing out the detail – it almost jumps out at you. This is a particularly effective technique for achieving detail vision.

To encourage following, a strong contrast has to be provided between the object that needs to be followed and the background. For this purpose, a device known as a 'shadow box' can be used. This is a long narrow box placed lengthwise, with a fluorescent light shining behind opaque glass. Face shapes and other designs can be cut out of heavy black paper, and then put on to short sticks to make a type of puppet. These puppets can then be passed in front of the shadow box, at close range to Mary. The light in the box will make the puppets stand out much more than normal, thus giving Mary a chance of being able to follow them as they slowly move across the light.

The pupillary reflex, following, and detail vision are the critical stages of visual development, and most attention needs to be directed at these levels. They are the essential foundations upon which the more sophisticated visual functions build. If Mary reached the point where she could follow and had very good detail vision, she would have achieved a functional level of seeing. Her vision should then continue to follow the normal pattern of development, provided she is given lots of things to see and appreciate, and thus can use her newly acquired function.

Hearing

Work should begin on Mary's hearing at the same time as an attempt is made to develop her vision, as different parts of the brain can be treated in conjunction with each other. As with blindness, some cases of deafness are caused by an injury to the brain. In Mary's case, the part of her brain that controls hearing has also been affected. If this part of her brain can be appropriately stimulated, there is a possibility that she may begin to hear.

Although Mary shows no response to noises of normal volume, a sudden, very loud noise produces a reflexive response – the startle reflex. Thus, she is at the lowest level on the auditory column of the Sandler-Brown profile. She has only a very primitive response to sound, but as with the pupillary reflex, it provides something to build on. Stimulation has to be started at this low level, by exposing her to lots of loud, sudden noises. The noises need to be very loud, and should last just two to three seconds. There should be five to ten seconds silence in between each noise, and each auditory session should last two minutes, with a variety of noises used – although only one type of sound should be made at a time. The session should be repeated 20–30 times each day. The sounds should be made within a close range, but from different directions, so as to encourage the later development of localization.

If these initial attempts are successful, Mary should begin to show more response to sound – her startle reflex may become stronger, and she may react to softer noises. Her awareness of the sounds around her may begin to develop, and she may eventually become wary and frightened of loud noises. At this point, instead of just loud sounds, Mary should be exposed to a wide variety of everyday sounds so that she can learn to understand what these noises mean – the appreciation of these sounds is an important step towards understanding words. At the same time, she should be taught to localize where the various sounds are coming from – this can be achieved by making sure the sounds are made from different directions. Finally, with constant exposure and careful instruction, she should begin to understand the spoken word.

Feeling

Mary shows almost no response to tactile stimulation. However, with a strong stimulus such as pinching, a slight reaction is noticed. She does not feel this painful stimulation nearly as much as she should, but at least she feels something. Thus, the initial tactile program for Mary would involve lots of vigorous stimulation – using things like a vibrator, brush, or strong massage and contact with the hands. As well, hot and cold objects should be used to teach her temperature differentiation. The tactile session should last for two minutes, and should be repeated 20–30 times each day.

If Mary begins to respond to these stimuli, work can begin on the next level of tactile development – the appreciation of light touch. Softer materials, such as silk and cotton, can be used in conjunction with, and in contrast to, the stronger stimulants. All these sensations should also help to develop body awareness.

It can be seen very clearly that, even with someone as severely brain injured as Mary, a treatment program providing appropriate sensory stimulation can be designed in accordance with how these senses develop in normal children. One advantage of such an approach is the relative ease with which these techniques can be applied. No fancy pieces of equipment are required – all that's needed are such things as whistles, bells, bright lights, vibrators, and brushes. As well, these techniques can be successfully carried out by parents in their own homes.

The same developmental concept needs to be applied to the treatment of Mary's motor functions – movement, speech and hand use. However, the development of these functions has to be approached in a different way to the sensory pathways.

It is possible to deal with each of the sensory functions in isolation. For instance, you can give direct visual stimulation without any interference from the other sensory pathways – you can still achieve constriction of the pupils, even if the child is deaf and insensate. At the lower levels of development, the way information is received through one sensory pathway is not affected by what is or isn't being received through the other pathways.

Such is not the case with motor development. In the early stages of growth, the three motor pathways are intimately involved with each other – this is especially true in the case of severely brain injured children such as Mary. Remember, movement is the key that helps unlock the brain. With Mary, her initial motor development is almost entirely dependent on achieving some kind of movement. Until she can go forward on her tummy, or hands and knees, it is extremely difficult for her to make significant progress in speech or hand function.

With brain injured children not as affected as Mary, the principles of normal development are more easily applied to the treatment of motor disabilities. Take the case of a child who is unable to walk: initially, an attempt should be made to incorporate into the treatment program the developmental stages that normal children go through on the way to walking. Attention should be directed to teaching the child to move on his tummy, then on his hands and knees, before trying to teach him how to stand and walk. You don't need to show a seven-month-old how to stand, as this occurs later, once their balance and coordination are sufficiently developed – as the child crawls around on his tummy and then on his hands and knees, his brain is gradually being developed until it is ready to deal with standing. Therefore, the same procedure should be followed with brain injured children, along with the attempted elimination or restriction of any undesirable or uncontrolled movements that may interfere with the higher levels of development.

The same applies to speech. An infant does not just suddenly begin to talk when he is twelve months old. First he has to go through all the preliminary stages – babbling, experimenting with sounds, learning to make word-like sounds, and then eventually words. The same process has to take place with brain injured children. A five-year-old who has never spoken cannot be expected to come out with words appropriate for his age when he first starts to talk. Instead, he has to go through the same developmental stages as a baby.

Penelope Leach[3] discusses this concept in relation to mentally retarded children who acquire speech late and then improve slowly, at the same time following the normal sequence of speech development:

In practical terms, it is unfortunate that this long-drawn-out language learning, within a normal, but usually much briefer, sequence, is not more widely recognized. All too often, a child of six or seven whose language development is equivalent to that of an eighteen-month old infant is 'written off' as being incapable of further language improvement. Even under ideal circumstances such a child would never catch up with his more fortunate peers. But if only he could continue to be given the kind of verbal help which is automatically offered to an eighteen-month infant, he would almost certainly continue to improve until he reached adolescence. And that might mean he would end up with a verbal age equivalent to a normal eight- or nine-year-old rather than equivalent to that of a toddler.

Again, the same principles apply to the development of hand function. A baby learning to reach out first makes very crude attempts, but with constant practice, and reinforcement, this skill gradually becomes more refined. A brain injured child learning to reach out has to follow this same pathway – his first attempts will be uncontrolled, just like a three-month-old baby, but he cannot be expected to reach perfectly without first learning to refine his movements. Lots of opportunity for simple reaching for large objects needs to be provided, before more difficult tasks can be attempted.

Thus, 'you have to walk before you can run' is advice even more relevant to brain injured children than to those developing normally. You cannot put a roof on a house without first laying the foundations and putting up the walls. Taking the child through the normal developmental sequences is, in effect, laying the foundations for future development.

CHAPTER THIRTEEN

Sometimes You Have To Start at the Beginning

IN CASE you are wondering, we have not forgotten about Mary. After talking about all the things that could be done to try and improve her sensory problems, we did not pursue the development of her motor abilities. Instead, we discussed children with less severe problems, as they better demonstrated the point being made. But for children like Mary, motor problems require special attention – that is why this issue is being dealt with in a separate chapter.

If you remember, we said that Mary's initial motor development was primarily dependent on the establishment of meaningful movement. If some kind of independent movement could be achieved, it should help to develop her speech and hand function, as well as being progress towards getting her to walk.

But Mary is three years old, and has never moved by herself in her life. And it appears unlikely that she will ever do so unless something can be done to help her. This presents a problem in itself because, since she has never moved, her brain has never felt what movement is like. All movement, although a function of the motor system, begins as a sensory input. The brain first learns what a particular movement *feels* like. Then, through repeated exposure, it learns how to control and purposefully use this movement. A lot of this initial learning takes place when a normal baby is lying on his tummy on the floor, as the brain feels and eventually controls the random reflex actions of the limbs that take place in this position.

However, Mary, and other severely brain injured children like her, usually miss out on this valuable input in two ways. Firstly, they are not often put down on the floor, as this is thought to be an unsuitable place for them. Instead, they spend a lot of time either lying or sitting. Secondly, as a result of their brain injury, the reflexive movements that are so prevalent in normal babies are often severely restricted. As well, there may be muscle tightness or weakness that prevents a normal range of limb movement. So, even if they were placed on their tummies on the floor, they do not have the right sort of movements to experiment with. However, despite the limitations that are present, these children should still be put on the floor some of the time, so that at least they can learn something about their body and about movement.

It may be difficult for you to imagine movement as first being a sensory input – that you initially have to feel the movement before it can be learnt. Probably the easiest example to relate to is the process of learning to drive a car that has a manual gear change. No matter how much theoretical instruction you are given about what is involved, the learning doesn't really begin until you get behind the wheel and try for yourself. In the beginning, it is almost impossible to coordinate the clutch and accelerater movement, and many 'bunny-hop' starts will result. But with practice you learn what the movements involved *feel* like, and eventually they become automatic. Your brain learns how much pressure to apply to each foot, and when this pressure should be applied or released.

So, imagine what it must be like if your brain has never felt any kind of movement. Although we know that Mary first has to learn to crawl on her tummy, and hands and knees, before she can learn to walk, it is not as simple as telling her to get down on the floor and do these movements. Her brain is not yet capable of this, so we have to start right from the beginning.

Her brain has to be taught what it *feels* like to move. Seeing that she can't do this by herself, it has to be done for her. Somehow, the proprioceptive information about movement has to be put into her brain.

One way of doing this is by a technique called 'patterning'. This involves moving the body through the same pattern of movement that an infant uses when he crawls on his tummy or up on his hands and knees. When an infant first begins to move on his tummy, he usually does so in a 'homolateral' pattern, with each side of his body working separately from the other. As he turns his head to one side, the arm and leg on that side bend into a flexed position, while the arm and leg on the other side extend or straighten out. When he turns his head, the limbs change position, with the arm and leg on the side to which the head is now turned flexing, and the limbs on the other side extending.

As the infant moves around more, and achieves better control over his movements, he usually changes into a 'cross pattern'. This is a more sophisticated movement, and involves coordinating the opposite sides of the body. It is also a more productive movement pattern, requiring less effort, but at the same time producing a smoother, more controlled movement. As the head turns to one side, the arm on that side bends into a flexed position, and the leg extends. The arm on the opposite side extends and the leg flexes. As the head turns to the other side, the opposite movements occur in each limb.

Seeing that we have to start right at the beginning with Mary, the homolateral pattern should be used first. This involves lying her face down on her tummy on a table. As she is only small, the patterning can be done with three people, but for older children five people may be necessary. With three people, one person moves the head, and one person is needed on each side of the table, moving the arm and leg on that side. As the head is turned to one side, the arm and leg on this side are bent to approximately 90 degrees at the shoulder and the hip, and the arm and leg on the other side are taken down straight (see diagram page 101). The head is then turned, and as this happens, the arm and leg on the side to which the head is turning are bent, and the arm and leg on the other side are straightened.

The patterning should be done in a nice steady rhythm, usually for five minutes duration. It is of utmost importance that the movement is well coordinated, so that the correct information is put into the brain.

If Mary begins to move by herself, her movements should become more coordinated, as a result of the continuing input from the patterning, and the practice and experimenting that she does by herself. At some point, the cross pattern needs to be introduced to replace the homolateral pattern – the exact time of this changeover varies with each child.

With the cross pattern, as the head turns to one side, the person on this side of the table bends the arm up and straightens the leg, while the person on the other side straightens the arm and bends the leg. As the head is turned to the other side, the arm on this side is bent up and the leg straightened, and the arm on the other side is straightened while the leg is bent. Again, this should be done in a slow, rhythmical movement (see diagram page 102).

Patterning is the initial attempt to put information concerning

Homolateral Pattern
3-man team

Start: In UP position and as the UP side (position 1) moves down, the DOWN side (position 2) moves up, in rhythm, as at position 3

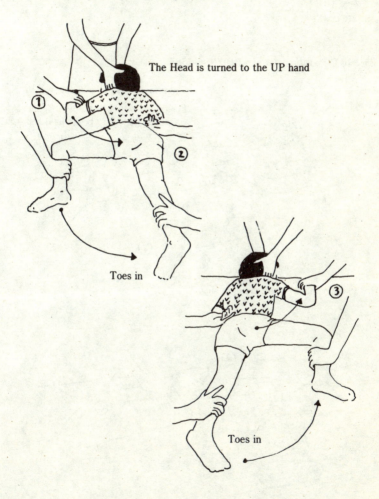

The Head is turned to the UP hand

Toes in

Toes in

movement into the brain. Of course, it is not as good as getting the child to do the movement himself, but for children who are unable to move, and whose brains have never felt what movement is like, it is necessary to start right at the beginning and provide this information for them.

Cross Pattern
3-man team

Start: In UP position at 1 and DOWN position at 3

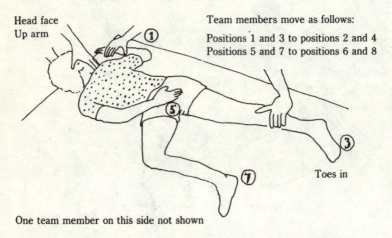

Head face
Up arm

Team members move as follows:

Positions 1 and 3 to positions 2 and 4
Positions 5 and 7 to positions 6 and 8

Toes in

One team member on this side not shown

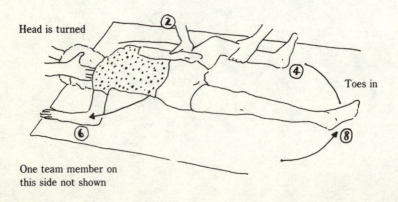

Head is turned

Toes in

One team member on
this side not shown

CHAPTER FOURTEEN

Input and Output

FOR the human brain to function correctly, three basic components are required – the input, processing, and output systems. If there is even a slight malfunction in any of these systems, the performance of the brain can be drastically affected. An understanding of the importance of each of these systems is essential if the brain is to be successfully treated following injury. Perhaps this can be best understood by looking at a situation that most people can relate to.

Nearly everybody has at least once, if not a hundred times, touched an object that was painfully hot. Hopefully, this object was released before any serious damage occurred. But for such action to have taken place, each of the three systems mentioned must have worked correctly. When the object was touched, information was immediately sent to the brain via the *input* system, which in this case was the tactile pathway. The message sent was that the object was dangerously hot. This was received and acted upon by the *processing* system in the brain, which then sent out the appropriate instruction: 'release the object' to the *output* mechanism – the hand and arm. This whole process took only a split second, for any longer would have meant serious injury to the hand.

Imagine what would have happened if any one of these systems was not working properly. If there was a tactile problem which prevented the person from detecting heat and pain, the object would have been held, with the person oblivious to the damage being done. If there was some kind of breakdown in the processing system, the message may not have been received, it may have been incorrectly interpreted, or either the wrong message – or no message at all – sent to the output system. If there was something wrong with the output system, such as spasticity or paralysis of the hand or arm, then even if the right message was sent out, it may not have been received or acted upon correctly.

Thus, what may seem like a simple action actually involves a complicated chain of events, with each component needing to function correctly for the desired response to take place. It is by this input-processing-output system that the brain operates in its everyday activities. It continually receives information from the environment, and, to the best of its abilities, responds appropriately to this information. Every second of every day, even during sleep, the brain receives input from both the internal and external environment which has to be continually acted upon.

To ensure that the' processing system in the brain can operate efficiently, the input system has to supply it with sufficient information about the environment. This system comprises the sensory pathways – vision, auditory, tactile, taste and smell. All these sensory inputs cannot be interfered with in any way without adversely affecting the performance of the brain.

The output system involves the motor pathways of the brain – mobility, speech and hand function. Not only do these have to operate unhindered, but also their performance has to be continually monitored.

The monitoring of motor output is in turn done by the input system. The sensory pathways pick up the results of motor performance from the environment. For instance, in the example of touching the hot object, the information was received and acted upon, but the correct action also required the monitoring of the initial motor response. This was done by the visual and tactile pathways – by seeing and feeling that the object was no longer being held. Without this input, it would not have been possible to know if the correct evasive action had been taken.

This complete input-processing-output-monitoring system is known as the 'feedback loop', and is explained in the diagram on page 105.

Most of the learning that occurs in the brain takes place via this feedback loop. Look at the example of throwing a ball at a target: if you throw the ball and miss the target, this information is fed back into the brain via the visual pathway. It tells the brain how the ball missed – if it was too short, too high, low, or whatever. Working on this data the brain will then try and modify the performance. The processing system will send a new set of instructions to the motor system, which then acts accordingly. This procedure will continue until the skill is mastered, or performed to the person's best ability.

The Feedback Loop

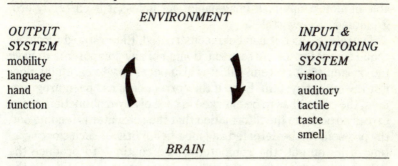

ENVIRONMENT

OUTPUT SYSTEM	INPUT & MONITORING SYSTEM
mobility	
language	vision
hand	auditory
function	tactile
	taste
	smell

BRAIN

Once the correct throw is made, it needs to be continually practised until the brain learns what is involved, and what needs to be duplicated in subsequent throws.

This skill, or any other for that matter, cannot be learnt unless the feedback loop is operating correctly. For example, if the lights in the room were turned off immediately after you threw the ball, you wouldn't be able to see where the ball went, and therefore it would be impossible to tell how close the ball was to the target. The brain would not receive any feedback to work upon, and it would be extremely difficult to master the skill.

Another good example of what happens when the feedback loop is disrupted is trying to talk to someone who is listening to music through stereo headphones. If you have ever done this, you will have noticed that the person always speaks much louder than is necessary. This is not premature deafness caused by all that loud rock music they have been listening to, but rather because the headphones prevent them from monitoring their own speech – they cannot hear how loudly they are talking. This is the reason why someone with a severe hearing loss often talks too loudly or with limited inflection. Not only do they have difficulty in correctly hearing the words and sounds that have to be reproduced, but they also cannot correctly hear their own attempts at speech. As a result, they are unable to make the necessary adjustments in terms of tone, volume and articulation.

In this respect, the human brain operates in a similar way to a computer, for a computer also utilizes the principle of the feedback loop. In the final analysis, a computer is only as good as the data that is programmed into it. You can build a billion dollar machine, capable of almost any task imaginable, but unless it is correctly programmed, it is worthless.

Therefore, once it has been constructed, the first and foremost requirement for the correct functioning of any computer is to have the proper input system. But it is also necessary to carefully monitor the output system. Even if the correct data has been programmed, the output has to be checked in case of any malfunction. If any errors do occur in the information that the computer is feeding out, the problem can be detected and modified. Without such close scrutiny of its output, the computer would continue to produce the incorrect material, without any knowledge of its error. This is the same type of feedback loop that governs the performance of the human brain.

To ensure that the brain works efficiently, the integrity of the feedback loop has to be maintained. Therefore, the input system – the five sensory pathways – has to provide all the necessary environmental information. As well, the output system – the three motor pathways – has to correctly carry out the messages received from the brain. In turn, the input system has to closely monitor motor performance.

Following brain injury, the feedback loop has broken down at some point. Therefore, an attempt needs to be made to try and locate the breakdown, repair the damage, and restore the loop.

The performance of the output system depends to a large degree on how well the other systems are working, as it is the end result of the information being correctly received and processed. Thus, this system is more difficult to reach. But the input system is more easily manipulated by external control, because it is possible to alter the quality and quantity of the environmental stimulation reaching the brain. As well, sensory input has a much greater effect on motor performance than would be expected. Given this, the sensory pathways into the brain need to be looked at more closely.

CHAPTER FIFTEEN

The Five Senses –
You Can't Live Without Them

W E SEE, hear, feel, taste and smell the world, and it is only through these pathways that the brain receives information from the external environment. Each of the five senses is essential for the proper working of the brain. Imagine what your world would be like if any of these senses malfunctioned. Most people equate sensory input – especially the senses of vision and hearing – with pleasure. Their initial reaction to the idea of sensory breakdown is to think how dreadful it would be if they could not see or hear the world.

However, there are more drastic consequences of such a breakdown than just the loss of aesthetic pleasure. For instance, the ability to perceive danger is solely dependent on sensory perception, primarily through vision and hearing. As well, sensory deprivation can actually be detrimental to the brain itself.

Imagine being faced with the prospect of having to give up four of your five senses. Which one would you choose to keep? Most people usually give the same answer to this question. The first two senses they are prepared to surrender are taste and smell, closely followed by tactility. Although these senses are pleasurable, they don't really compare to the joy gained from seeing and hearing. Thus, the choice comes down to which gives the most pleasure – the eyes or the ears. Almost everybody decides to retain vision, for they would rather see a silent world than hear a black one.

But which sense is the most important from a neurological standpoint? As satisfying as it is, you can survive quite well without vision – look at all the blind people in the world. You can survive without hearing too – look at all the deaf people. You can certainly survive without taste and smell, as these are the two least important senses.

The one sense you cannot live without is tactility. A totally insensate person – someone unable to feel any kind of pain or light touch, and without any body awareness – is probably suffering from a very severe brain injury. With such a complete loss of tactile input, it would be impossible to have any greater function than that of a severely brain injured person.

You simply cannot manage without tactility. If you cannot feel, most motor functions are impossible. Let's look at a couple of examples: if you sit for too long in an awkward position, your leg sometimes 'goes to sleep'. What actually happens is that, as a result of the sitting posture, some of the blood supply to the leg is restricted, temporarily shutting down some of the nerves in that area. Try as you might, you cannot walk on this leg, because the essential information regarding the position and state of the limb is not getting through to the brain. Without this vital input, the brain loses control of the leg. According to the concept of the feedback loop, a specific breakdown has occurred in the tactile pathway, rendering the leg useless until the blood supply normalizes and the sensation returns. If the telephone happens to ring while you are sitting there waiting for your leg to 'wake up' you will discover that this process cannot be hastened, and you probably will have to hop over to the phone on your good leg.

A similar situation may have happened to you at night while sleeping. If you were lying awkwardly on your arm, the circulation would have been restricted, sending your arm to sleep. Like most people, you would have woken because of the discomfort this causes. What a strange situation – you wake up because your arm is asleep, then you have to lie there until the arm wakes up before you can go back to sleep again!

A trip to the dentist is another example of the effects of interference to the tactile pathway. The pain killing injection works well in reducing the pain, but the numbness that persists afterwards causes problems. Answering the telephone can be embarrassing, as you are afraid that the person on the other end of the line will think you have a speech impediment. Worse still is trying to eat a bowl of soup at a restaurant, only to be told that some soup is dribbling out of your mouth!

In all of these situations, there has been no physical damage to the leg, arm or mouth, and yet their functions have been severely affected. Thus, any interruption to the flow of tactile input to the brain can have quite a profound effect on motor performance.

But, the effects of tactile deprivation are not just restricted to the motor functions of the brain. In fact, totally unrelated areas can be adversely affected – as demonstrated by a fascinating study done in Canada in the early 1960s[1]. A group of twenty-two male university students was placed in a deprived tactile environment for seven days. This was achieved by prolonged immobilization – they were placed in coffin-like boxes that were lined with a thick layer of foam rubber cut out in the shape of a human figure. The feet and arms were put into restraining devices to stop any movement, and the head was also restrained. They were unstrapped and allowed to sit up for fifteen minutes at meal times, and were allowed to get out for one hour in the afternoon, during which time they went to the bathroom and were given various tests. They were also unstrapped for nine hours during the night, but were not allowed to sit or stand up.

Since only the effects of tactile deprivation were being tested, care was taken to ensure that the students received other types of stimulation. They could hear people moving about and talking, and they could listen to the radio whenever they wished. Various pictures were placed above them and changed from time to time, and the lights were turned out at night.

The subjects were given various intellectual and perceptual-motor tests before, during and after the experiment, and their brain patterns were measured by an electroencephalogram machine (EEG). At the end of the seven days, all the subjects who had been immobilized performed worse on all twelve of the intellectual tests given, than control students used for comparison who had not been immobilized. Also, their results on two of the five perceptual-motor tests showed significant impairment. An examination of the EEGs at the end of the study revealed that the immobilized subjects had a significant decrease in electrical output in the occipital lobe area of the brain.

Zubeck and Wilgosh (see note 1 above), the Canadian psychologists who conducted this study, felt that the results they had achieved were very significant: 'The study has demonstrated that reducing the level and variability of tactile-kinesthetic stimulation via immobilization can produce a disturbance of both performance and the electrical activity of the brain.'

These results were achieved even though the tactile deprivation was not as severe as the scientists would have liked (they felt that the results would have been even more convincing if a greater amount of deprivation was involved). All the subjects endured the week quite easily, indicating that it was not particularly stressful for them. The fact that significant results were still achieved – despite the deprivation being moderate – only further underlines the importance of tactile input to the brain.

The results of these intelligence tests on the immobilized subjects raise an interesting question. How is it that students deprived of tactile stimulation performed poorly on tests that had nothing whatsoever to do with tactility? None of the items on the intelligence tests were even remotely connected to sense of tactility, and yet the performance on these tests was adversely affected.

It is apparent from these results that a prolonged period of tactile deprivation affected not only the tactile part of the brain, but also had a depressing effect on overall brain performance, even to the point of decreasing its electrical output. Similar effects of generalized depression of brain activity have been seen in studies dealing with visual and auditory deprivation[2,3]. Although the functions of the brain are to a certain extent localized, with specific centres controlling individual functions, these centres do not operate in complete isolation from each other. Thus, as shown by the tactile deprivation study, interference to one of the sensory pathways into the brain also affects other areas of brain function.

Even more dramatic results are achieved if the deprivation involves all of the senses[4,5]. Zubeck, *et al.*, report on just two of the many studies that have been done on overall sensory deprivation. They state that in one study looking at the effects of prolonged isolation, approximately one third of the volunteers failed to endure such conditions for longer than four days. The effects of isolation and deprivation have been known for centuries, and the manipulation of the sensory environment has proven to be one of the most effective forms of criminal punishment.

Without doubt, one of the most severe types of punishment is solitary confinement. If you have ever visited an old gaol that was in use in the eighteenth or nineteenth century, your lasting impression of such an institution probably would have been the isolation of the solitary confinement cells. It is amazing that anybody survived being in such a confined area for just a day, let alone the months on end that some prisoners were subjected to. It's no wonder that even the most violent, unrepentant inmate often came out as gentle as a lamb after his time in solitary. As Zubeck and his colleagues state:

'One can only wonder about the possible physiological and psychological state of prisoners of war and others who, in the past, have been isolated for months or even years.'

Many brain injured children have been condemned to live in solitary confinement within their own bodies. As a result of their brain injuries, the sensory pathways have been seriously disrupted – especially in the case of severe brain injury. Such disruption literally adds insult to injury since interference to the sensory pathways can further damage the brain. A vicious cycle is created – as a result of the brain injury, the sensory input is disrupted; as a result of the disruption to the sensory input, the function of the brain is further hindered.

Although the consequences of sensory interference are known, as is the fact that brain injury can cause such interference, the importance of treating the sensory problems of brain injured children is sometimes overlooked. This is especially the case when the problem is related to the tactile pathway. It is relatively easy to detect if a child is blind or deaf as a result of injury to the brain. But major tactile problems sometimes go unnoticed. Take for example a child who is completely immobile, unable even to hold his head up. This absence of movement would naturally seem to be a motor problem caused by injury to the movement part of the brain. However, with close examination it often can be seen that such a child is completely unresponsive to any sort of tactile stimulation. You can pinch him quite hard, or even prick him with a pin, and yet he shows no reaction.

It's no wonder that this child cannot move. So bad is his tactile problem that he probably isn't even aware that he has legs and arms. You can't walk on your leg when it has 'gone to sleep'. Imagine what it would be like if your whole body was like that! Remember, Zubeck's work showed that adverse effects from prolonged immobilization occurred within just seven days – many brain injured children have been immobilized and insensate for *years*.

Such children have a two-fold problem: their lack of movement is not just a motor problem, for it also involves the sensory input into the brain – primarily the tactile pathway. Therefore, the treatment for these children has to be directed at both movement and tactility. In the initial stages, most of the attention should be concentrated on the tactile problem, for until the child becomes aware of his body, he cannot move. Such treatment should involve lots of strong tactile input, such as a vibrator, body brush, loofah sponge, and body rub. It should be done in two-minute sessions, 20 to 30 times a day. Once the tactile problem begins to improve, more effort can be put into using the appropriate techniques to develop movement.

It was stated earlier in this chapter that interference to one sensory pathway can have an adverse effect on other areas of brain function, since each brain area does not work in isolation. Of the utmost importance to the treatment of brain injured children is the fact that the reverse is also true – if you *increase* the amount of stimulation reaching the brain through a particular pathway, you may also stimulate and enhance other areas of the brain. For instance, we have just seen that increasing the amount of tactile stimulation for an insensate, immobile child can also have a positive effect on movement. Improving the hearing of a child with a severe auditory problem will be a positive reinforcement for the development of speech, since language is largely dependent on hearing. Improving the vision of a child with a severe visual problem should help in the development of movement and hand function, seeing that vision obviously plays an important role in these areas.

The various parts of the brain do not work in isolation. Therefore, all the ways in which brain injury can manifest have to be closely examined to ensure that the pathways in and out of the brain are functioning correctly. If they are not, they should be treated appropriately. Particular emphasis should be placed on sensory input since any interference in this area can have a drastic effect on motor performance.

CHAPTER SIXTEEN

Frequency – Intensity – Duration – the Key

SO FAR IN this section, we have been discussing the important aspects of an effective treatment program – the need to establish and maintain the feedback loop by the use of appropriate sensory stimulation and motor opportunity.

But another critical factor has to be considered before we can go any further – the manner in which the various techniques should be applied.

Any treatment program is only as effective as the way it is conducted. Even the best techniques available would be unsuccessful if they were administered incorrectly. Thus, it is not just a question of what should be done, but also when and how often.

There are three basic principles that need to be considered in the practical application of any treatment technique. These principles are founded on perfectly sound neurological facts. It is likely that if you read the following statement to any neurologist, you would find him in complete agreement:

In order to increase central nervous system transmission – that is, to get more messages to and from the brain – you have to do three things to the stimulus provided. You have to increase its *frequency, intensity* and *duration.*

The three most important words in this book may well be – *frequency, intensity* and *duration.* They are the three most important principles upon which a treatment program is based. Even if you forget most of the things in this book, you must remember these three words!

Frequency, intensity and duration

You have to increase the frequency of the stimulus . . . You have to increase the frequency of the stimulus . . . You have to increase the frequency of the stimulus . . . You have to increase . . .

You HAVE TO INCREASE THE INTENSITY OF THE STIMULUS. YOU HAVE TO INCREASE THE INTENSITY OF THE STIMULUS. YOU HAVE TO INCREASE THE INTENSITY OF THE STIMULUS.

You have to increase the d-u-r-a-t-i-o-n of the stimulus – like we have just done.

The principles of *frequency, intensity* and *duration* have just been employed. The message was repeated often (frequency), the size of the print was increased (intensity), and the message was continually sounded (duration). In one hour from now, we are sure that most people will remember what they have just read, for the information has reached their brain in a more powerful way than normal. Frequency, intensity and duration of the stimulus is the most effective means by which the brain can learn.

Let's forget about brain injured children for the moment, and look at other aspects of life in which these three principles are employed. Take the case of a marathon runner. An enormous amount of time and effort has to be spent in building up the strength and stamina necessary for such an event.

In working out a training program, the first thing that the athlete has to consider is how far to go on each training run. To most of us, the idea of running twenty kilometres is frightening enough, but this is the bare minimum that the athlete has to achieve most times he goes out for a run. For instance, Robert de Castella, the famous Australian marathon champion, runs up to 220 km a week in training.

How often he trains is the next thing that the athlete must consider. Two or three times a week would be insufficient, as it needs to be a daily activity. Even if he ran very long distances, say 70 km three times a week, this would not be a good training program, as constant repetition is needed to build up the stamina required.

Once he had devised the ideal training program, the athlete would then have to estimate how long it would take to build his body and mind to the point where he could run the distance in a competitive time.

Such are the demands of marathon running that it is not something he could achieve in just a few months of training. Robert de Castella estimated that it took him two years of extremely intensive training to reach the point where he almost broke the world record for the marathon.

It can be seen that the whole training program for the marathon runner is based on the principles of *frequency, intensity* and *duration* – how far, how often and for how long he keeps it up.

All doctors know the importance of frequency, intensity and duration in respect to the correct use of medications. The way a drug is taken is as important as its actual contents. The proper dose has to be determined (intensity), as well as how often it needs to be taken (frequency), and over what period of time (duration). No matter how good the medication is, it will not be effective unless it is taken as prescribed.

These three principles also apply to the learning of any new motor skill. As any sportsperson will tell you, it is only with constant practice and repetition that a skill can be mastered, with the amount of practice time being much greater than most people would anticipate. Crossman[1] studied a group of women from the time they were first employed in a cigar factory until the time where they reached their peak performance in the manual task of cigar making – the point at which Crossman felt they had developed an engram of manual skill (an engram being a pattern of coordination required for a specific task that is firmly and completely programmed into the brain so that the task can be successfully repeated without any new learning being required). He found that it required *three million* repetitions of the task before the cigar makers achieved their maximal rate of performance.

Commenting on Crossman's findings, Kottke[2], a U.S. rehabilitation doctor, agreed that it required millions of repetitions of any single task for a person with normal coordination to reach their peak skill level. The comments of one of his colleagues with whom he discussed this are worth repeating:

I believe you. However, do not publicize this information. The idea that development of coordination requires millions of repetitions is so overwhelming that therapists will be too discouraged to try and develop coordination in their patients.

Kottke goes on to discuss how much repetition he feels is necessary for a skill to be perfected:
● Tens of repetitions produce testing and awareness of isolated performance by a coordination unit, but result in little retention.

- Hundreds of repetitions begin to create a faint and fragile engram which will fade quickly.
- Tens of thousands of repetitions form a fair engram in which speed and force can begin to increase.
- One hundred thousand repetitions result in significantly increased skill.
- Millions of repetitions are required to perfect an engram.

How do the three principles of frequency, intensity and duration apply to the treatment of brain injured children? In the next chapter, we will show how frequency, intensity and duration can be used when dealing with the most severe type of brain injury, and thereby with less serious problems. But, before examining a specific problem, a general comment needs to be made concerning the amount of treatment a brain injured child needs.

Given that frequency, intensity and duration are so critical to the success of a treatment program, obvious care should be taken to ensure that each child receives the correct amount of therapy. But, how is it possible to tell exactly how much treatment each child needs? Unfortunately, there is no scientific way of measuring a 'prescribed dose' of therapy. This is unlike the situation where a doctor needs to prescribe a particular drug, for the dose that is required has already been established as a result of scientific research carried out by the drug company.

If only it was so easy to determine how much therapy and stimulation each brain injured child needs. However, there are no manuals or reference books that can be consulted which will outline the exact type and amount of treatment a particular problem requires. There is no 'typical' case of brain injury, therefore there can be no standard treatment procedure.

If you took two brain injured children with similar problems and functioning at the same level, and you gave them exactly the same treatment, they would almost invariably respond differently. Although these children appear to have the same problem, it is impossible for them to have suffered identical brain injuries. We have already seen how incredibly complex the brain is, therefore the exact same type and amount of brain cells could not have been destroyed in these two patients. Thus, with even minor variations in the injury to the brain, they could not be expected to respond identically to the same treatment program.

Since there are no hard and fast rules, experience is the best teacher of how much treatment is best for a particular child. But at the same time, it is not possible to predict how each child will respond. This is one of the first lessons to be learnt when dealing with brain injured children – the extremely unpredictable nature of brain injury. Just as you think that your foresight is improving, along comes a child whose progress is completely contrary to what you would have expected.

One of the major problems in the treatment of brain injury is this inability to scientifically measure how much therapy is necessary. Depending on which treatment centre or therapist you go to, there will be a wide variation in the amount of therapy suggested. One of the most contentious issues concerning the type of treatment described in this book is that it involves a much more intense therapy program than most other organizations offer. Some people claim that this intense application of therapy is inappropriate, but we consider it to be vitally important.

The determination of how much therapy we prescribe for each child is a very individual matter. There are many things that need to be considered – the child's age, the severity and type of his injury, his health, the family situation, and any other relevant factors. The therapy program may vary from just one or two hours a day with a very young child or a child with minor problems, up to as much as eight hours a day with a severely hurt older child.

Take the case of a nine-year-old child who, despite the severity of his brain injury, has only been doing one hour a day of therapy – as is often the case in conventional treatment. In this situation, we would possibly advocate up to eight hours of therapy daily. Some people throw their arms up in horror at such a proposal, for to them it seems cruel to have to subject such 'unfortunate' children to so much therapy.

But these same people accept that a normal nine-year-old child needs at least six hours a day of therapy – for isn't this what he gets at school? Can you imagine what would happen if the government proclaimed that all nine-year-olds were only allowed to receive one hour of education a day? There would be widespread demonstrations, since most people feel that normal children need to spend all day at school to ensure their proper education and development.

However, when we suggest that a brain injured child of the same age be given an equal amount of stimulation and learning, the reaction is completely different. In fact, the brain injured child actually needs the attention more than a normal child, for if he is ever going to have a chance in life, he needs all the therapy he can get. But, since nobody really expects him to make significant progress, it seems unfair to subject him to so much treatment. After all, wouldn't it be better to just keep him happy, rather than making him work all day?

If it was true that a brain injured child could never improve, then it would indeed be cruel to carry out an intensive treatment program. But who can tell if he will or will not progress? And who can take the awesome responsibility of predicting that he won't improve, and therefore denying him therapy that may change his life?

Often these negative, sympathetic attitudes work completely against the child. Little chance is given by the doctors for the child to improve, so he receives only a small amount of therapy. As predicted, the child progresses poorly, thereby making the initial prognosis seem correct, as well as justifying the decision not to implement an intensive therapy program.

But wait a moment. How much of the lack of progress is due to the severity of the brain injury, and how much to the fact that little is done to treat it? It is a vicious circle – nothing much is done about the child's problem, therefore he doesn't progress; he doesn't progress, therefore nothing much is done about his problem.

Until now, it generally has been assumed that the absence of any real improvement in most severely brain injured children has been because these children are beyond help. Certainly, the poor results from conventional treatment observed over the years have done nothing to disprove this theory. So, with this kind of thinking prevalent, there seems little reason to institute intensive therapy programs for such children. In fact, until now an inverse relationship has usually existed between the severity of the brain injury and the need for treatment – the more severe the problem, the less reason seen for intensive therapy.

But, it should be the other way around. Severely brain injured children have the greatest need for intensive therapy, especially soon after the problem develops or becomes apparent.

The principles of frequency, intensity and duration are essential to the treatment of brain injury, particularly in the case of severe injury. We now need to look at how these principles can be practically applied.

CHAPTER SEVENTEEN

Coma – the Most Severe Brain Injury

UNLESS you have seen a person in coma, it is hard to imagine that a human being can be so totally unaware of, and unresponsive to, the outside world. But if you have, you will know what a devastating sight it is. It's hard to tell if they are dead, or just in a very deep sleep. No stimulus appears to be getting through, and it seems impossible to wake them.

The comatose state is not a disease in itself, but is the end result of a very severe injury to the brain. It can result from a strong blow to the head, asphyxiation, the ingestion of toxic substances, or any other severe insult to the brain. It can be a temporary condition, lasting just a few hours or days – in such cases, the patient sometimes wakes up spontaneously and recovers normal or near-normal function. But, all too often, it becomes a prolonged state of unconsciousness, with the associated danger that the person will suffer a severe loss of function if he does come out of coma. Worse still, there is no certainty that the patient will ever wake up, for the comatose state can become a permanent condition. For example, the longest coma on record lasted for thirty-seven years.[1]

What is the physiology of coma? Contrary to what may seem obvious, coma is not related to sleep. Before scientists became aware of the true nature of coma, it seemed logical to think of a person who couldn't be woken as being in a deep sleep. If you have ever tried to wake a person who is a heavy sleeper, you will have discovered how far removed some people can get from environmental stimuli during sleep. You may have even jokingly referred to this person as being 'unconscious' as you tried in vain to wake him.

Translated from its Greek origin, 'coma' actually means heavy or deep sleep. Thus, it was originally thought that after a severe trauma to the brain, the body went into a sleep-like state as a means of self-protection. However, research has now shown that this isn't so, as the state of consciousness or arousal is not controlled by the body's sleep mechanism. In fact, sleep and consciousness operate quite independently of each other.

Jouvet[2], a French neurologist, states that research into sleep has shown that stimulation of the sleep mechanism will cause an animal to go to sleep, but this is not a permanent or prolonged loss of consciousness, as the animal eventually awakens. Jouvet also mentions that other studies have shown that while damage to the sleep mechanism produces a state of prolonged insomnia, it does not affect the animal's ability to perceive environmental stimuli.

Since the brain area controlling sleep is not directly related to coma, it is necessary to try and locate the area or areas that are. Jouvet states that the comatose person's failure to respond to environmental signals may theoretically result from the following types of lesions, or injuries, to the brain:

1. A lesion of the sensory pathway that prevents external stimuli from reaching the integrating central structures of the brain (the brain areas responsible for receiving, processing and sending out information).

2. A lesion of the motor pathway that prevents a response to the stimulus.

3. A lesion affecting the integrating central structures.

Studies of animals have shown that a lesion of the sensory pathways in the brain stem does not lead to a coma[3]. As well, it is now widely accepted that a person who is unable to express a motor response because of damage to the motor pathways, can still receive complete environmental stimuli if the sensory pathways are intact. Thus, through a process of elimination, it can be seen that coma seems to be caused by lesions to the integrating central structures.

In humans, there are two integrating central structures. One is the Reticular Activating System (RAS), the area in the brain responsible for the maintenance of consciousness. The other is located in the frontal lobes of the cortex, and this acts as the cortex's integrating system.

The RAS is located between the spinal cord and the midbrain. It receives information from all the sensory receptors of the body – these receptors send their input along a bundle of fibres that course through the spinal cord and brain stem. They relay information to the RAS at many different levels. Once the information is sorted and analysed in the RAS, the appropriate messages are distributed to the various parts of the cortex in order to maintain a normal state of arousal and function. The RAS thus acts as a network relay station, receiving incoming signals and distributing them to the relevant brain areas.

The role of the frontal lobes in maintaining a suitable level of consciousness is somewhat different, for one of their responsibilities is to exert a general activating influence on the RAS. As such, the frontal lobes play a secondary role in the maintenance of consciousness. They help activate the activating system (the RAS). They also ensure that the cortex maintains a suitable level of function by modifying the state of waking so that the level of output is appropriate to what is required at any particular time.

The difference between these two integrating systems is shown by the contrasting effects displayed when each system is destroyed. Destruction of the cortex, and thus the frontal lobes, results in a loss of all learning ability. However, reflexes such as the pupillary and startle reflexes remain, and the animal can be aroused from its sleep. On the other hand, destruction of the RAS completely abolishes learning ability and severely impairs reflex responses, even though the cortex is still intact. The eyes are closed, the pupils constricted, there is no response to auditory and tactile stimulation, and the brain wave pattern shows that the cortical activity consists entirely of slow waves that remain unchanged by all sensory stimuli, with the exception of smells[4,5]. As would be expected, an injury that simultaneously affects the two integrating structures has the most profound effect on the brain function, characterized by a complete absence of perception and reactivity, and by total cerebral silence on the EEG reports.

Unlike most other types of brain injury, quite a lot is known about the actual mechanism of coma. Thus, it could be expected that, with this more precise knowledge, the treatment of coma would be more advanced. Unfortunately, this is not the case. In fact, parents of a child in coma encounter many of the same difficulties and frustrations that are experienced by parents of other brain injured children.

The first problem is that of definition, for there seems to be a considerable amount of confusion in this area. There is no commonly accepted definition of coma, as can be seen by looking at some of the many that have been presented:

- The inability to obey commands, to utter recognizable words, or to open the eyes.[6]
- The inability to establish intellectual contact.[7]
- A state of unconsciousness from which the patient cannot be aroused.[8]
- The absence of clinical (or paraclinical) signs of appreciation of the environment. (See note 2 above.)

Of all the definitions presented, we feel the following is the most appropriate: *A pathological state of unconsciousness from which the patient has not yet reached arousal.*[9] This implies that coma arousal can be achieved and therefore *should* be attempted. This issue will be taken up in the next chapter.

But first the orthodox approach to the treatment of coma needs to be closely examined. The intensive care stage of this treatment is nothing short of magnificent, for modern medicine does a marvellous job in saving the lives of many traumatically injured patients. However, our concern is with the patient who leaves the intensive care ward in a stable condition, but without showing any signs of coming out of coma.

In 1965, A. K. Ommaya[10], a neurosurgeon in the United States of America made a frank assessment of the situation at that time regarding the treatment of coma patients. He said: 'Considerable advances have been made in recognizing and treating the surgically remediable complications of head injuries, such as depressed fractures, intracranial haematomas of various types, and infections. However, we have not achieved equally significant progress in understanding cerebral concussion. The management of closed head injuries remains empirical, and the resultant mortality, although less than it was 20 years ago, is high. More importantly, the quality of survival after severe head injuries could be improved.'

It would be safe to say that Ommaya's statement is till true today. Although the surgical and intensive care techniques have continued to improve, the treatment of patients with closed head injuries (those not needing surgery) remains unsatisfactory. The 'quality of survival' is still in great need of improvement.

In 1977, a group of scientists released the results of a study they had done regarding the outcome of patients who were in coma following head injury[11]. They studied patients in three countries – Scotland, the United States of America, and the Netherlands – and noted their state of recovery six months after injury. In the Glas-

Table 5: Outcome of patients who sustained coma from head injury

	Glasgow (428)		Netherlands (172)		Los Angeles (100)	
Dead	221	52%	89	52%	49	49%
Vegetative state	8	2	1	1	5	5
Severe disability	34	8	9	5	18	18
Moderate disability	71	17	26	15	14	14
Good recovery	94	22	47	27	14	14

gow section of the study, 428 patients were observed. Of these, only ninety-four, or 22 per cent, made good recovery. Seventy-one (17 per cent) were classified as having moderate disability, thirty-four (8 per cent) were severely disabled, eight (2 percent) were in a vegetative state, twenty-one (52 per cent) died within the first six months. Similar results were obtained in the other two countries, as can be seen from Table 5.

From this study it could be concluded that – at least during the first six months – only a small number of patients seem to make a good recovery from head injury that is severe enough to cause coma.

Why such poor results? One reason is that if the brain injury is severe enough to result in coma, it is likely to make spontaneous arousal and recovery of function extremely difficult. But this is only part of the answer, for it also has to do with the post-intensive care stage of treatment. Given that *spontaneous* recovery is made difficult by the severity of the injury – in fact, the patient remains in coma because spontaneous arousal has not occurred – it would seem logical that every attempt should be made to try and 'wake' the patient.

However this is often not the case. If a patient is transferred out of intensive care still in a coma, it is usually thought that there is little that can be done to shorten the length of the coma. Therefore, a wait and see approach is adopted in the hope that the patient will eventually wake up. Routine hospital treatment is administered to take care of the patient's basic needs, and usually regular physio-therapy is given in the form of 'range of motion' exercises to help prevent muscle and joint tightness from becoming too severe. However, in most cases little therapy is given that is specifically designed to try and arouse the patient.

Such a passive approach can be partially justified by the fact that some patients do eventually come out of coma spontaneously, and the hope with each patient is that they will be one of these lucky ones. But, what happens to those who are not so fortunate, and whose coma goes on and on? In these cases, they cannot wake up by themselves – that's why they remain in coma. So why just sit around and wait for something that may never happen?

This passive approach is similar to someone being put in a completely dark room, and, instead of searching to see if there is a light switch, they just sit there assuming there isn't one and hope that someone will eventually come and illuminate the room. If the person stuck in the darkened room was to search for a switch and find one, there would be no guarantee that the light would work – but at least it would be worth trying.

There are inherent dangers in not doing everything possible to shorten the length of coma. First, the brain injury that caused the coma may be so severe that it will prevent the patient from achieving natural arousal. In such a case, the comatose condition may continue indefinitely if a wait and see attitude is adopted.

Second, there is statistical proof that the length of coma has a direct effect on the patient's chances of eventually regaining consciousness. The longer the coma continues, the less chance the patient has of being aroused, and the greater is the probability of residual problems being present if the patient does eventually come out of coma.

Such a relationship was shown in a study by United States researchers, Stover and Zeiger[12]. They looked at what happened to forty-eight patients, all under twenty years of age, two or more years after a traumatic head injury that had caused a coma lasting more than seven days. Thirty had spent less than thirteen weeks in a coma, and of these, all but one were able to walk at the time of the follow-up evaluation. In stark contrast, of the ten who came out of coma at or after thirteen weeks, only two had achieved independent walking.

During the first three months of coma, Stover and Zeiger found no direct correlation between the duration of coma and resultant functional recovery. However, they did observe that if the coma lasted longer than seven days, it usually resulted in some kind of permanent physical and/or mental impairment. Although nearly all of the patients who were in coma less than three months ended up walking, most still required supervision during activities of daily living, and some needed aids to assist with their walking. Of those in coma longer than three months, it seemed that independent living could only be expected in very unusual cases.

A close analysis of the statistics compiled in the previously mentioned three-nation study (see note 11 above) also shows that the first months after the beginning of a coma are the most critical. According to the authors of this study, if progress is going to be made, most of it occurs in the first three to six months. Of those in the category of good recovery after one year, 60 per cent had already achieved this level in the first three months, and 89 per cent by six months. Of those classified as moderately disabled at one year, 62 per cent were in this category at three months, and 92 per cent by six months.

English researchers Galbraith, Jennett and Raisman[13] offer a fascinating hypothesis in an attempt to explain why recovery from coma, if it happens at all, seems to occur primarily in the initial months after the injury. They compared the rate of collateral sprouting (described in Chapter 6) that occurred in rats following surgical brain injury, with the rate of recovery from coma due to head injury in humans.

With rats, they found that collateral sprouting is very rapid for the first month after injury. It then gradually approaches completion (i.e. complete or near-complete restoration of the original connections) over the next two months.

The researchers then made a comparison to the rate of recovery seen in humans, using the data gained from the three-nation study. They made the observation that the recovery rate in the human patients was similar to the rate of collateral sprouting that occurred in the rats. In conclusion they state: 'Whether the process observed in rats has any relevance to functional recovery after brain damage in man is unknown, but it seemed of interest to compare the time scale of these two biological events.'

With the risk of placing too much emphasis on what was really only a scientific observation of two similar, but possibly unconnected events, this issue should be looked at more closely. One conclusion that could explain the similarity between the two rates of recovery is that the process of collateral sprouting is, to some degree, involved in the humans' recovery from coma. Following this line of thought, it then seems possible that both recovery rates stopped at around the same time because this was when the collateral sprouting slowed down or stopped.

If these conclusions are correct, and remember that they are only based on an hypothesis, this provides strong evidence for the need to start treatment as soon as possible after the beginning of coma. If collateral sprouting does occur in humans after brain injury, and if it only continues for a short period of time, then the early stage of coma is the time to institute an intensive therapy program designed to achieve coma arousal. This appears to be the time that the brain is actively undergoing attempts at self-repair, and it is possible that in this dynamic state, it would be more receptive to attempts at stimulating it into action. Perhaps the combined effects of external and internal endeavours to achieve restoration of function would be more conducive to reaching the desired result.

Thus, it is quite obvious that the length of coma is critical to the patient's eventual outcome. The fact that a patient does not reach arousal at an early stage indicates that the injury suffered by the brain is quite severe – the more severe the injury the less likelihood there is of early arousal. But, apart from the severity of the injury preventing arousal, the extended period of coma is in itself making arousal more difficult.

The state of coma adversely affects the function of the brain. It creates an obvious case of severe environmental deprivation, because it acts as a barrier that prevents all or most environmental stimulation from reaching the brain. The effects of sensory deprivation have already been discussed, and since this deprivation in a coma patient is usually quite severe and prolonged, it must have a detrimental effect on brain function.

As well, coma results in a generalized depression of brain activity, as shown by the decreased electrical activity that is a feature of the EEGs of most coma patients. The work of Eccles[14] has shown that at cellular level, depressed function decreases the ability of the cells to transfer information. He states: 'Prolonged disuse has a deleterious effect on the potency of the synapses.'

The fact that coma patients are almost completely immobile (apart from the range of motion exercises that may be given) raises another critical issue. The work of Zubeck and Wilgosh[15] concerning the effects of prolonged immobilization, discussed earlier, is very relevant to the person in coma. These researchers noticed adverse effects on performance and brain electrical activity after just seven days of immobilization – extremely mild deprivation compared to that suffered by a comatose person. Zubeck and Wilgosh saw the relevance of their work to patients in a state of prolonged immobilization, and stated: 'Adverse psychological effects may occur if appropriate measures to stimulate bodily activity are not taken' Thus, frequent range of motion and other body exercises are vital not only to help prevent severe joint and muscle tightness from occurring, but also to give the brain essential tactile-proprioceptive input.

Perhaps you can now understand just how detrimental coma is to the function of the brain. It combines the effects of severe sensory deprivation with almost total immobilization. It is little wonder that coma can continue for long periods of time, and that those who eventually regain consciousness are often left with residual problems, for coma is indeed the most severe form of brain injury.

The patient in coma is in a helpless state. If his condition does not quickly improve, it gets much worse, since the longer the coma the less chance of arousal, and the greater the probability of being left with severe disabilities. There are too many risks involved in passively waiting and hoping for the coma patient to 'wake up'. Instead, a way has to be found to arouse him, and it must be done as quickly as possible.

CHAPTER EIGHTEEN

Coma Arousal – Restoring the Feedback Loop

' JOSHUA fought the battle of Jericho and the walls came tumbling down.' So go the words of an old religious song. Joshua,
faced with an impenetrable wall around the city of Jericho, was able
to bring the wall down by angelic intervention and the combined
voices of the children of Israel.

The condition of coma acts like the wall around Jericho as it
forms a seemingly impenetrable barrier between the brain and the
environment. As established in Chapter 14, the feedback loop has
to be maintained for correct brain function. Any interference to the
input system can have drastic consequences.

For a patient to be aroused from coma, a way has to be found by
which stimulation can reach the brain, with the ultimate goal of
restoring the feedback loop. The wall has to be knocked down, for
as long as it remains the patient will stay in coma. How much stimulus gets through the wall will largely determine how far the patient
comes out of coma.

But, without divine intervention and the combined vocal power of
the children of Israel, how on earth can the brain be reached?

With every normally functioning human being, there are only five
direct ways in which the brain can be stimulated. The five tools at
our disposal are the sensory pathways – vision, hearing, touch,
taste and smell. These are the only ways that the brain can receive
information about the world around it. This is how a baby first
receives messages from its environment, and it is how we continue
to relate, every second of every day, to a constantly changing
world.

In a normal situation, stimulation sent along any of these pathways activates the brain, providing that the stimulus is strong
enough. Is it possible that these direct pathways into the brain can
be utilized in an attempt to achieve coma arousal? The simple fact is
that this is the *only* way it can be done.

The sensory pathways are the only means of reaching the brain. But, with a coma patient, these pathways are apparently closed and it seems that no matter what input is applied, it gets no further than the barrier formed by the coma – bringing us back to the original problem. But not quite – for we now know there are five *potential* ways of reaching the brain.

These sensory pathways are not working while the person is in coma, but that is not to say they cannot be made to work. During coma, a normal level of sensory input is usually insufficient to reach the brain – that's why a coma patient shows no reaction to his environment. But if the sensory input can be manipulated, it may be possible that the five sensory pathways will become the saving grace of the person in coma. For this to happen, the principles of *frequency, intensity* and *duration* have to be employed. To show how this can be done, each sensory input needs to be looked at separately.

Vision

As stated in Chapter 10, the lowest level of visual function is the pupillary reflex, the constriction of the pupils in response to light stimulation. How well the pupils constrict is largely dependent on the strength of the light. If a low intensity light is used, such as a torch with flat batteries, the pupil constriction of a normal person will be incomplete. If a strong light is used, the constriction will be very rapid, with the pupils becoming very small.

If you shine a torch light into the eyes of a coma patient, you may get no response at all, even if it has new batteries. But this does not necessarily indicate a total absence of visual function. It may be the equivalent of what happens with a weak light and a normal person – the light is not strong enough to activate the pupillary reflex because the complete stimulation has not reached the brain.

Most people would assume that a coma patient in this situation has no visual response. But what would happen if a stronger light was used? Is it possible that the increased intensity could stimulate the desired response? With many coma patients, if a strong enough light source is used, it *is* possible to make the pupils constrict. The light may have to be very strong, say 150 watts, and the constriction may be sluggish and incomplete, but nonetheless, what an achievement! Constriction of the pupils means that the barrier has been broken through, and the brain reached. It may only be for one second, the time usually prescribed for shining such a strong light into the eyes, but the critical factor is that the brain has been stimulated.

What would happen if the light was repeatedly shone into the patient's eyes, many times a day, with the pupils constricting each time? Whenever the light was turned on, the barrier would be penetrated, and it is possible that a pathway into the visual part of the brain would begin to be established. Just shining the light once or twice a day, even if it was strong enough to constrict the pupils, would be like Joshua's lone voice trying to knock down the walls of Jericho. It can only be done with the combined effect of frequent effort.

Even if the correct intensity of light was used repeatedly, little progress would be made if it was only continued for a week or two. To achieve the desired result, keeping in mind the magnitude of the task at hand, it is essential that this stimulus be kept up for many weeks and months.

Therefore, first of all the correct *intensity* of light has to be found – strong enough to create the pupillary reflex. This then has to be applied with the proper *frequency* – many, many times during the day. Lastly, both of these principles have to be carried out over a suitable *duration* of time if an alternate visual pathway is to be established in the brain.

It is not possible to set out an exact visual program here, as each patient has to be individually assessed before the appropriate treatment can be determined. However, the following routine is fairly typical: the light usually needs to be at least 150 watts, and the visual session should be done in a dark room. The light is held 40–50 cms (15–20 inches) from the face, and is shone into the eyes for one second, and then switched off for five seconds, and then repeated. One visual session consists of 20 flashes of one second on, five seconds off, and this session is repeated approximately 25 to 30 times each day. Where possible the eyelids should be lifted to expose the pupils. If this is impossible, shining the light at the closed eyes should still elicit a response, but in this circumstance, an even stronger light should be used. If a patient is in such a deep coma that the pupillary reflex cannot be created even with a very intense light, this procedure should still be carried out in the hope that the continual stimulation may start to make inroads into the brain.

As the visual pathway, hopefully, starts to develop, the patient will begin to open his eyes, or they will be open more often. At this point, work may need to be done on developing the ability to follow and see detail, depending on how much visual ability returns. Bright pictures and posters should be put around the bed, and the patient shown familiar pictures and photographs. It is usually impossible at this early stage to assess how much the patient can see, so stimulation should be provided in case he is beginning to recognize things around him.

Auditory

The startle reflex is the lowest level of auditory function, and therefore the point from which to start with a coma patient.

As with the pupillary reflex, the critical factor in creating the startle reflex is the intensity of the stimulation. A patient in coma may not respond to noises that would startle a normal person, but if a loud sound is made, it is often possible to produce a startle response. This may involve banging two old saucepans together, blowing a loud whistle, or ringing a bell – the important thing is to make a loud enough noise that will get the desired response.

If the startle reflex is created, this means that again the barrier has been broken and a stimulus registered in the brain. If this can be repeated often enough, chances are that it will start to open up an auditory pathway into the brain. The principles of application are exactly the same as with visual stimulation – of prime importance is the intensity of the sound, which must be strong enough to get some sort of response, and then used with the correct frequency and duration.

The way in which these sounds are made is also of critical importance. If you have ever been exposed to a constant noise, you will be aware how it is possible to 'turn off' the sound – even if it was irritating at first. The brain has the ability to filter out, to a certain degree, constant noise. But it cannot do this to irregular noise, that is, to sounds that occur without any pattern. For most people, this type of noise is extremely irritating.

If the auditory stimulation for the coma patient is just a constant noise, there is a possibility that this filtering process could diminish the effect. Therefore, it is best for the noise to be made for two or three seconds, followed by five to ten seconds of silence, without any pattern being used. This auditory session is usually done for two minutes at a time, and repeated 20 to 30 times a day. If the patient is in a hospital or nursing home, the staff and other patients won't take too kindly to the disturbance, so some modifications need to be made. It is possible to record the sounds on an audio cassette, and then play them through a set of headphones at high volume. In this way, no one will be disturbed – except, hopefully, the patient.

Although a coma patient may not appear to be responding to noise, it is still possible that he can hear and understand everything around him, including the conversations of the hospital staff and those people visiting him. Failure to recognize this can have drastic consequences. Take the example of Patrick, a patient who was in coma, but eventually regained consciousness. Although he was in a prolonged coma, Patrick could hear and understand everything around him. He remembers very clearly a particular day that his mother was visiting him – the doctor came into his room, and assuming Patrick could not hear anything, he proceeded to try and convince Patrick's mother that it would be best to turn off the respirator and let him die peacefully. Imagine how you would feel, lying there and hearing all of this, without being able to respond in any way. Patrick said that it was sheer hell, for he had absolutely no means of telling his mother that he wanted to live.

Seeing that it is often impossible to determine if a coma patient can hear and understand, it is best to assume they can, and talk to them quite normally, especially about things they would be interested in. Also, situations like Patrick's should never be allowed to happen. No negative comments should be made within earshot of the patient, nor should anything be said that may upset him. Favourite music can be played through headphones, and a television should be on some of the time showing his favourite programs. Even if he is not able to hear or understand, such a procedure is not harmful, and it will ensure that he is surrounded by appropriate stimulation when this faculty hopefully develops.

Tactile

Given the choice between being tickled and being pinched, most people would prefer the tickling, as it certainly is the more pleasant sensation. Unfortunately, a coma patient cannot be given such a choice. He needs both types of stimulation, but most importantly, lots of the rough stuff. There is a much greater chance of crossing the tactile barrier and getting through to the brain if a strong intensity of stimulation is applied. With a strong stimulus, a response is often seen from a person in coma, either a grimace or some kind of body movement – a sign that the message has reached the brain.

Strong tactile stimulation can be achieved by deep pressure massage, pinching and slapping (firmly given, but not to the point of bruising), and by the use of a vibrator, loofah sponge, and body brush. This should be done to all parts of the body, and applied firmly enough so that it would be unpleasant if you were doing it to yourself. You have to bother the person in coma if you are going to get through to his brain. Light touch will not do this, although it is still a good stimulation to give in contrast to the more intense input. Other types of tactile activities that should be included are temperature variations using hot sponges and ice, and proprioceptive input (body awareness). Since the brain is denied the feeling of movement as a result of immobilization, this has to be given to the coma patient. Range of motion exercises, which move all the accessible joints through their full range of movement, are appropriate for this purpose, and they should be done for five to ten minutes at a time, 10 to 15 times a day.

Do not be afraid of applying strong tactile stimulation to a coma patient – providing it does not cause any damage to his body – as this is the best way of getting through. In this situation, being gentle is not necessarily being kind.

Taste

Seeing that every available means of stimulating the brain has to be utilized, the senses of taste and smell become very important when working with a coma patient. Again, the most critical factor is the intensity of the stimulus. If a strong taste is given, it is likely to cause a reaction, such as grimacing – a sign that something has reached the brain.

Some tried and tested tastes that often get reactions include vinegar, lemon juice, mustard, soy sauce, chili, and strong salt and sugar solutions. These can all be applied quite simply. A tiny amount on a cotton bud placed on the tongue, or just inside the mouth if the jaw is kept tightly closed, is usually sufficient to cause a reaction. In addition, pleasant tastes previously enjoyed by the patient should be included.

The taste session usually lasts two minutes, with a variety of tastes being used in each session, and this is repeated about 15 times a day. If possible, the tongue should be wiped with a moist cloth or cotton bud between tastes, to remove the previous stimulation. Special care should be taken to avoid making the patient gag, but this is rarely a problem, seeing that only such a small amount of the substance is applied via the cotton bud.

Smell

Given that the intensity of the smell is most important, some effective smells include peppermint oil, eucalyptus oil, garlic, strong perfumes, rubbing alcohol, and undoubtedly the most effective, spirits of ammonia. Only a small amount needs to be placed on a cotton bud, which is then passed under the patient's nostrils. The patient may grimace or attempt to withdraw, proof once again that the brain has been stimulated.

The smelling session usually lasts two minutes, with a variety of smells being used in each session, and is repeated about 15 times a day. As well as strong stimulants, pleasant smells should also be used, especially any that the patient previously enjoyed.

In addition to the sensory stimulation and the range of motion exercises, vestibular or balance stimulation needs to be given to the coma patient. This will provide input to the balance areas of the brain, and is another effective means of helping to achieve arousal.

If the patient's physical condition permits, he should be rolled from side to side on a soft mat, with care being taken to ensure that his arms and legs do not get caught in an awkward position. If this is impossible, then at least some gentle rocking from side to side in the bed should be instituted. This vestibular work should be done for two to five minutes at a time, and should be repeated about ten times a day.

It should be clear now how the principles of frequency, intensity and duration apply to the treatment of the coma patient. It virtually amounts to a continual bombardment of the brain through the sensory pathways. Of the three principles, intensity is the most critical, but the other two are not far behind in their importance. The program should be built up to at least eight hours a day, and should be carried out for six to seven days a week. Such is the severity of the problem that there is no easier way.

Family, friends and volunteers should be directly involved in the treatment program. In fact, they should be the primary therapists. As can be appreciated from the description of the program, it is relatively easy to carry out, and can be very effectively and efficiently done by these people once they have been carefully taught. Realistically, they are the only ones in the position to devote the attention that is necessary each day, for the hospital staff simply cannot spend so much time with just one patient.

The psychological bonding that occurs is also very important. Carrying out this program is obviously an expression of great love and dedication towards the person in coma. Such emotions are often felt by the patient, and help to give him the inner strength and determination not to give up. The power of love in these situations is just as important as any stimulation that is being given through the sensory pathways.

Careful counselling, as well as special support, should be given to those implementing a coma arousal program. At no time should it be thought that this is something they must do, for it should be a voluntary action, based on the belief that they could cope with the physical and emotional demands it would put on them.

In our experience, many parents of children and young adults in coma are anxious to begin any sort of treatment program that may help to arouse their loved one. It is so frustrating for them not knowing what to do. Day by day, they often sit beside their child in the desperate hope that he will wake up. But all they can do is helplessly watch their imprisoned loved one who is unable to free himself. Giving these parents something positive to do is often as good therapy for them as it is for their child.

If Joshua, with a lot of physical and spiritual help, can make the walls of Jericho come tumbling down, then surely an attempt can be made to do the same to the 'walls of coma'. In doing so, the feedback loop will be restored, thereby creating the best possible situation for the proper working of the brain.

At least it's worth a try, for what is there to lose?

CHAPTER NINETEEN

Traumatic Brain Injury

'HEAD INJURY' is the term generally used to describe brain injury resulting from a blow to the head, a car accident, a fall, or any other traumatic injury affecting the head and thus the brain. However, this is a most unsuitable label as it is much too vague. A lacerated forehead could be said to be a head injury, even though it may not have affected the brain in any way.

'Traumatic brain injury' is a much more accurate description in these cases, for it describes the real problem. As well, it encompasses the types of injury to the brain that are not the result of physical damage to the head, such as drowning, asphyxiation, and electrocution. This diagnosis can therefore be used to describe a person whose previously normal function has been adversely affected by a trauma-related brain injury. While it affects people of all ages, our interest is with children and young adults.

At the beginning of this book, we dealt with parents' reactions to the realization that their child had been born with some kind of brain injury. In some ways, it may be even more difficult for parents who see their normal child struck down by a traumatic insult to the brain. Having a perfectly healthy, active child suddenly turn into someone who is helpless and almost alien must be a shattering experience. Here is how Sydney mother, Gemma Giardini, describes the experience of almost losing her son, Kevin, in a drowning accident, only to be left with a child incapable of any function:

At two-and-a-half, Kevin was the brightest, most adorable, affectionate little scallywag in the world. He used to bring me flowers that he'd sneak from next door's garden . . . he knew I loved flowers. And what a chatterbox – he'd never stop talking!

You couldn't have wished for a happier, more normal kid. I used to love watching him run around, full of the limitless energy that toddlers have. He was interested in everything. Maybe that was why it was so hard coming to terms with his accident. One minute he was a lively, loving, normal child, and the next minute he was severely brain injured. Bang. It was as sudden as a kick in the teeth. There was no warning, no gradual deterioration of his condition.

There are absolutely no words to describe the horror that gripped my heart after the accident. It was a profound, overwhelming shock. The grief my family and I felt seemed to suck us into an abyss, a black hole in space. And at that stage, we could see no light anywhere.

Kevin had strayed into a neighbour's yard and fell into their swimming pool. He must have been in there for several minutes before we realized he was missing. After frantically searching, we found him in the pool, floating face down. He wasn't breathing, and attempts to resuscitate him didn't work. An ambulance was on the scene within minutes and I can still picture the para-medics trying to revive him – but Kevin wouldn't take the oxygen.

He was pronounced clinically dead when we arrived at the hospital. It's hard to describe the terror I felt at the thought of losing him. I loved him so dearly and the thought that he might die was more than I could possibly bear. I didn't care how badly hurt he may be, I just wanted him to live. I prayed and prayed as the medical staff desperately tried to revive him in intensive care. They managed to save his life, but he went straight into a coma and stayed like that for several days. I can clearly recall a doctor taking me aside and saying: 'Only a miracle will save him now'. I prayed for that miracle. He did live, and I thank God for that. But he was a completely different child when he finally came out of coma. This Kevin was as rigid as a board, had no speech, no apparent sight, hearing, sense of touch or smell, and no motor abilities whatsoever. My husband and I felt helpless and shaken to the very core of our being. We just couldn't believe or accept that this had happened to us. We couldn't believe it was really true – but there was no escaping the terrible reality of the situation.

The hospital doctors offered no advice, no help – they didn't even suggest counselling, and I suppose we were too dazed to ask for help on our own behalf. They told us that there was virtually nothing we could do for Kevin, that we should not expect any improvement in his condition. They told us to take him home and love him and cope as best we could. If we weren't able to cope, we should put him in an institution and try and resume a normal family life, they said.

I found this insulting. You don't just stop loving your child because he is sick or brain injured. You can't just shut him out of your life and forget he exists because he is no longer 'perfect'. We *didn't* stop loving Kevin. If anything, we loved him *more*.

We desperately wanted to try and do something, anything, to help our little boy get better. We did not just want to sit back and accept that there was nothing that could be done, to accept that our previous, dearly loved son would spend the rest of his life as a living vegetable.

But that was the picture that was painted for us. The days ahead seemed completely devoid of hope. The medical staff made it very clear – Kevin was a child with no future.

Following any traumatic brain injury, there is always the possibility that spontaneous recovery will occur. However, as with the coma patient, there is no guarantee that this will actually happen. Therefore, it is not a wise practice to adopt a wait and see approach. Instead, intensive treatment should be instituted as soon as possible after the injury has occurred.

If spontaneous recovery is going to take place, it usually happens within the first six months. If it hasn't occurred by then, it is unlikely to happen after this time. Unfortunately, if a patient does not make significant natural progress (improvement not related to specific treatment), this is often interpreted as a sign of permanent injury, and in these cases, little emphasis is put on intensive therapy – in fact, if there is no response, the treatment is often scaled down. But, the fact that the patient has shown no meaningful progress in the first six months is not necessarily an indication that he will never progress. Rather than decreasing the intensity of the treatment, it should be *increased*, for what other chance does the patient have? An intensive therapy program should be carried out for at least twelve months before any assessment can be made regarding the future of the patient.

There is one question that almost all parents of traumatically brain injured children ask, and it goes something like this: 'Seeing that my child was normal before, will it be easier for him to regain the functions that he has lost?' The answer to this question is closely related to the nature and severity of the brain injury. In the case of severe injury, many of the cells that were controlling the various functions have probably been destroyed, and if this is so, a patient in this situation is unlikely to be any better off than someone injured from birth. If it is only a mild injury, the loss of cells will not have been so large. In this case, it may be easier to restore function – by re-using superseded pathways, and by expanding the existing network of undamaged connections.

Regardless of the severity of the injury, the principles involved in working with traumatically brain injured patients are basically the same as for patients injured from birth. In a way, both situations are similar – a certain portion of brain cells has been destroyed, but there is still an enormous reserve of unaffected cells which have to be stimulated into action. The means by which these cells may be reached is also the same – via the use of appropriate developmental stimulation and opportunity, given with the correct frequency, intensity and duration.

For instance, in the case of a fifteen year old who has been totally immobilized as a result of a car accident, the ultimate objective would be to get him moving again, hopefully to the point of walking. Even though he is fifteen, he needs to be treated in accordance with his neurological rather than chronological age, seeing that he is functioning at a very low level. The most logical way to teach him to walk is by taking him through the same developmental stages that a baby experiences on the way to walking – tummy crawling, crawling on hands and knees, cruising, and standing independently. As well, weight bearing in the supported near-upright position, on a device known as a tilt table, may need to be incorporated. Apart from walking, the same developmental principles would need to be applied to the attempted restoration of any other functions lost.

There are both positive and negative aspects to working with a traumatically injured patient, compared to working with a child injured from birth, especially if the trauma patient is a young adult. A three-year-old, injured from birth, may be quite a way behind his peers, but not as far as the eighteen year old who has suffered an almost total loss of function after crashing his motorbike. As well, obviously it is physically more difficult to work with a big strapping eighteen year old than a child of three.

Motivation may be a big problem with a teenager or young adult. He may be frustrated and depressed about his present condition, and may have adopted a defeatist attitude, to the point of refusing to cooperate with therapy. Also, if the frontal lobes were affected by the insult to the brain, aberrant behaviour problems may develop which could make the therapy more difficult to administer.

Depending on the severity of the injury, and the time elapsed since the accident, physical problems may have worsened to the point where they could hinder the therapy program. Especially in the case of someone in coma, muscle and joint tightness can set in very quickly and what starts out as simply a symptom of the brain injury then becomes a major problem in its own right. This problem will be exacerbated in patients who have received inadequate post-trauma care.

On the positive side, we have already said that if the patient has suffered a mild injury, he may be able to utilize the already developed parts of his brain that remain unaffected by the injury. This would not be the case in someone injured from birth.

If the patient has retained some or all of his intellectual capacities, as is often the case, this may be a tremendous advantage. If he understands the nature of his problems and realizes the need for intensive therapy, he should be a very motivated and willing worker. In such cases, great care needs to be taken to fully explain the purpose and rationale behind what is being done. Like most people, he would probably find it much easier to work if he knew the reasons for what he was doing. Even though his speech may have been affected, this has no bearing on his understanding. Unfortunately, such patients are often spoken down to, or ignored, as their lack of speech is interpreted as an absence of understanding. This only makes their problems all the more frustrating.

Perhaps the biggest advantage of working with traumatically injured patients who are older and have good understanding, is that when they begin to make progress, their awareness of their improvement usually serves as a tremendous source of self-motivation. This helps a great deal in keeping them willing to carry out the hard work that is required. It is extremely difficult, if not impossible, to rationalize with a three-year-old that although he might not enjoy it too much, the therapy is good for him, and therefore he should do it.

Perhaps the best example of how this can work is shown by the attitude of Michael, a thirty-year-old patient from Brisbane. Michael worked extremely hard for five years, diligently carrying out a six- to eight-hour therapy program, six days a week. Happily, he made excellent progress – he learnt to walk again, his speech and eyesight improved dramatically, and he is now completely independent – something his parents were told would never happen. Asked what motivated him to keep working so hard for so long, his answer was so simple and yet so wise: 'It kept on making me better than I was.'

CHAPTER TWENTY

Who Controls What?

SINCE THE human brain has billions of parts and an incredibly complex network of connections, it must also have an extremely well established system of control. Such control needs to be clearly defined and rigidly adhered to, otherwise chaos will reign supreme. Luxuries such as democratic rule and freedom of speech are not allowed, as there is a firmly entrenched hierarchy of power. The cerebral cortex is dictator and supreme ruler. It sits on top of a throne – the brain stem – and sends out orders which are unquestioningly obeyed by the lower echelon of cells. The only time that the cortex loses its absolute control is during potentially life-threatening situations, for at these times the lower, reflexive parts of the brain assume control until the danger passes.

The cortex enjoys all the comforts of being an autocratic leader – once it has made a decision, all the hard work involved in carrying it out is done by those below it. The cortex's job is to make a rational assessment of all the information available, and then give the appropriate commands. Once the instructions are sent out, it becomes the task of the lower brain areas to organize and coordinate all the necessary parts of the body so that the correct action can be taken.

However, like some of history's less successful dictators, the cortex is sometimes not happy with just handing out directions, and instead tries to run the whole show. If this occurs, disorder usually follows, for the cortex ventures into foreign territory. It was designed to make decisions, not carry them out.

Learning to drive a manual car is a good example of what can happen when the cortex gets involved where it shouldn't. In Chapter 13 we looked at this example to show how movement is first a 'feeling' that the brain learns to control and reproduce. We now want to look at what is involved in mastering this skill, and why it is so difficult in the beginning.

Anyone who has learnt to drive will no doubt remember just how impossible it seemed when you first got behind the wheel. There was just so much involved! To change gears you had to gradually take your foot off the accelerator, while simultaneously depressing the clutch – and you had to make sure that these two movements were coordinated. While the left foot was down on the clutch, you had to shift the gear stick into the correct position. Once you had done this, the left foot had to be lifted off the clutch, while the right foot was put back down on the accelerator, with split-second timing and perfect coordination. At the same time, you had to carefully watch where you were going, and be aware of what was behind you – and all of this while steering correctly. But most importantly, you had to stay relaxed. Stay relaxed! With so many things to worry about, how on earth could you?

The reason why everything seemed so difficult was because you were 'driving with your cortex'. Ordinarily, the cortex just tells you which direction to follow as you drive along – but in this case, it was directly involved with all the complicated movements required when driving a car.

In defence of the cortex, this was not really a case of it over-stepping its authority. When any new activity is learnt, the cortex has to be involved as the lower parts of the brain, primarily the midbrain, haven't yet learnt what to do. This is why new skills are difficult to master in the beginning. With sufficient practice, the right information is programmed into the lower brain areas, and they learn what the movement *feels* like – and the task seems almost second nature. Once this has happened, it becomes the sole responsibility of the midbrain to reproduce what is required on subsequent occasions, and the cortex returns to its rightful role of sending out instructions – it is no longer involved in the mechanics of the task. For instance, when was the last time you consciously thought about what you were doing when you were driving? Did you remember to tell yourself to put your foot on the clutch and take the other foot off the accelerator as you changed gears? Hopefully not, otherwise you would still be driving like a learner.

We tend to take everyday activities for granted, especially things that seem easy to perform. But, if you stop to analyse exactly what is involved in even the simplest tasks, you begin to appreciate just how important the lower brain areas are. To demonstrate this point, let's look at what would happen if it were possible to put the midbrain to sleep, thereby leaving the cortex to carry out activities as well as give the orders.

Take the example of reaching out, picking up a pencil, and holding it above your head – normally a very easy task to perform. Since the midbrain is out of action, the first thing that the cortex has to do is analyse what muscles will be involved in the movement required. Even before reaching out can begin, the muscles in the hand, arm and upper torso have to be in proper relationship to each other, with some needing to be tense, others relaxed. As well, the shoulder, elbow, wrist and finger joints have to be in proper relationship to each other, as do the various ligaments that hold these joints in correct alignment.

All of these extremely complicated calculations would have to take place before you could begin the movement, so as to prepare the body for action. But, this would be only the beginning of the cortex's worries. Since all of these relationships change with every micro-second of movement, the cortex would continually have to stop everything to make sure that all the muscles, joints and ligaments were in their correct positions.

With so much for the cortex to think about, it would take forever to accomplish the required task – if it was in fact possible. And yet, under normal circumstances when the midbrain is functioning correctly, it takes just a matter of seconds to reach out, pick up a pencil, and hold it above the head – without any thought whatsoever being given to the intricate coordination required. All the cortex needs to do is give the command, and this is then carried out by the midbrain.

In some cases of brain injury, the cortex gets involved where it shouldn't, and performance can be adversely affected. Athetosis is a particular type of brain injury which results in a severe motor problem, highlighted by a great deal of uncontrolled, flailing movement. Many athetoid children are extremely bright, and although often unable to communicate verbally, they can function very well intellectually. In other words, the athetoid's cortex (the thinking part of the brain) continues to operate effectively – the problem lies in the midbrain (the movement part of the brain).

One of an athetoid's biggest difficulties is that the more his cortex gets involved in a motor activity, the worse his performance gets. If you ask an athetoid to reach out and pick up something, the more he thinks about it, and the more you remind him of what is involved, the harder it is for him to do what is asked. As he thinks about what he is doing, the cortex sends more and more messages to an already confused area of his brain, making everything even more chaotic. Of course, this becomes very frustrating for him, for it is virtually impossible to control his well-meaning cortex.

And yet, parents of athetoid children all tell the same perplexing story. They have observed situations where their child performs much better than he normally does when he is not thinking about what he is doing. For instance, he may be watching television or listening to a conversation, and without realizing it, he reaches out and picks something up almost perfectly. In this situation, the cortex is already preoccupied, so the child operates primarily with the midbrain. Without the extra confusion from the cortex, he can gain some control over his movements.

The appropriate roles of the cortex and midbrain need to be understood and applied to the treatment of brain injured children. The cortex is primarily the thinking part of the brain, and the midbrain is directly involved in coordinating and controlling the movement patterns of the body, therefore it seems logical that many of the movement and motor problems caused by brain injury result from injury to the midbrain area. Thus, it is this part of the brain that needs to be treated if these motor problems are to be rectified. It also follows that a problem which has originated in the midbrain cannot be successfully treated if the treatment is directed at the cortex.

For instance, take the case of a child with an articulation problem. If you work with him in front of a mirror and make him aware of how to place his tongue and lips correctly to form the proper sound, he may be able to do it perfectly – provided he keeps concentrating on the mirror. In fact, it may be possible in these circumstances for him to make the correct sound repeatedly. But, as soon as he goes outside and starts playing with all the kids in the neighbourhood, you will hear him going back to his old way of speaking. In the therapy sessions he is fine, but there seems to be little carry-over.

The reason is quite simple – in therapy he is learning to talk with his cortex. As soon as he leaves the room, his cortex forgets all about reminding him where his lips and tongue should be, for it has more important things to do. When was the last time you thought about your lips and tongue while you were talking? Probably never, as this is an automatic function of the midbrain. This part of your brain learnt what was involved a long time ago when, as a baby, you made all the normal baby sounds, thereby learning what the lips and tongue should do. Also, at the same time you probably did a lot of crawling and creeping, which helped to firmly establish the motor pathways and teach the brain about the intricate control of movement.

Parents of a child who walks with a slight limp may have thought of his problem as an inability to pick up his toes on his 'bad' foot as he steps. They may have explained to the child that for normal walking, a heel-toe action is required – the heel strikes the ground first, then the toe. They may have then devised what seemed to be an ingenious way of teaching their child to walk in this fashion. They walked around with him, and each time he was about to step with his bad foot, they said: 'pick your toe up'. As long as the child concentrated on the instruction given, and provided the problem was not too severe, he may have been able to pick his toes up and walk correctly. If the parents kept walking around with him, whispering the magic words in his ear, he may have continued to perform well.

But, there is one catch – the parents need to be there all of the time to remind him to pick his toes up. If they are not, or if he is distracted by something, he will immediately go back up on his toes and start limping again. The voice in his ear is treating his cortex, and as soon as it stops, the control of the movement returns to its rightful place, the midbrain. The problem recurs because, instead of treating the problem area, the cortex is used as merely a temporary detour.

Why is it that you never have to teach a normal child how to pick his toes up when he first starts to walk, and yet he does it in perfect heel-toe fashion? His midbrain learnt all about this action when he was on the floor learning how to crawl and creep. When a baby crawls on his tummy, a lot of the propulsion comes from pushing off with the feet, a movement that requires digging the toes into the ground. As the leg bends up, the toes are also brought up, so that they are in the best position for propulsion. Think of the number of times that an infant crawling around on his tummy has made this movement – perhaps thousands. By the time he gets up to walk, the action of picking the toe up as the leg bends has been so well programmed into the brain that it has become an automatic response requiring no conscious thought. The midbrain has been taught this movement during the early stages of development without the cortex being directly involved. Even though a child may have missed the stage of tummy crawling, he still probably would have experienced the reflexive movements of his knees and toes coming up as he was lying on his tummy on the floor or in his cot. Therefore, his midbrain would have learnt what it feels like to 'pick your toes up'.

When treating the motor problems of brain injury, an attempt must be made to improve the function of the midbrain, by exposing it to the repeated feeling and experience of the correct movement patterns. This can usually be achieved through the use of appropriate developmental activities and stimulation. For instance, the process of patterning that was described earlier is a good example of this principle. Patterning is the language of the midbrain – it teaches that part of the brain what correct movement feels like.

Thus, it is necessary to respect the hierarchical power structure that exists within the brain. Each area is responsible for vital functions, some more apparent than others. The cerebral cortex is indeed the master of the brain, but no master can function properly without its loyal subjects. As well, all levels of control have to be considered when the brain is treated, with the treatment being directed at that level of the brain where the injury lies.

CHAPTER TWENTY-ONE

Females Aren't the Only Ones with Instincts

MALES have long been accused of dominating and controlling most aspects of society, but there is one female domain that, it would seem, has remained safe from this ubiquitous masculinity. Who has ever heard of male instincts? It seems that whenever human instinctive behaviour is discussed, it is always in reference to females. Males, apparently, are devoid of intuitive thought or behaviour. So, for all those males who may feel inferior in this area, we are about to present *one* example of male instinct. One small step for man . . .

At times, most members of the animal species seem to be deliberately rough with their young. A mother dog rolls her puppies endlessly across the floor with her nose. A mother cat will pick up her kittens by the scruff of their neck, shake them about, and throw them around. It is curious to note that, in these lower animal forms, it always seems to be the female who treats the young in this way.

As the young grow older, they appear to incorporate these types of activities in their play. For instance, they may endlessly roll each other around, sometimes quite vigorously. Although such behaviour may seem rough, the baby animals have a wow of a time.

In sophisticated animals, such behaviour still exists, but with one interesting difference. It is now the male of the species who takes on the role of exposing the young to this apparent rough handling. A female gorilla is usually very gentle and protective of her babies, but the male becomes 'King Kong' as he spins the baby above his head and throws him around.

This same kind of behaviour can be seen in humans. Approaching bed time, mothers usually begin to calm baby down by gentle rocking and singing. But fathers seem to have a different idea of how to get baby ready for bed. Because they often have limited time with their child, this is one opportunity for fun and games. Suddenly the

147

baby becomes a human helicopter and goes flying through the air. Shrieks of joy – from both father and child – are heard coming from the bedroom. Of course, after all this the baby is no longer interested in going to sleep, and mum is left with the job of calming him down. Does this sound like a familiar story?

Most fathers seem to have an uncontrollable urge to pick up their baby and throw him around. This is not restricted to bedtime only, for often in play the same thing occurs. Why do they do this? It is not something they are taught, and it is certainly not encouraged by the child's mother, who half expects baby to come crashing down on to the floor at any moment. Most fathers say that they do it because the child likes being thrown around. Certainly, most babies do like it. In fact, they can never seem to get enough. But dad could not have been sure that *his* child would enjoy it the first time, so why did he do it?

We believe that it is an instinctive pattern of behaviour for animals to occasionally be rough with their young. In lower forms of animals this is the responsibility of the mother, but for some reason this changes in higher animals, and the father assumes this role.

Being moved rapidly in space stimulates and activates the balance mechanism in the brain – the part of the brain that is responsible for the maintenance of correct balance and equilibrium. If the child is not exposed to rapid body movement and different body positions during development, the maturation of this brain area could be adversely affected. A child needs to experience this rapid movement, as he later has to cope with it during everyday activities.

This is why fathers swing their babies. This is why three and four-year-olds spin themselves around so much that adults feel sick just watching, and why they hang themselves upside down on the playground gym equipment for so long that it seems as if all the blood will rush to their head. All of these activities are a necessary part of development, because they stimulate the balance area of the brain, thereby helping to ensure its proper growth. Babies can't do these things for themselves – that's where dad steps in. But with older children, these activities are incorporated into their play.

Perhaps we need to take a look at the way in which the brain maintains a correct relationship to the outside environment – a function known as 'spatial orientation' – to better understand why these instinctive spatial activities are so important. The way the brain reacts to spatial *dis*orientation best illustrates how spatial orientation is maintained.

A very simple way of feeling what it is like to be disorientated is to spin yourself around rapidly. Most people cannot do this for very long, as they soon feel nauseous and have to lie down until the spinning sensation stops. The brain is unable to cope with the rapid spinning, and the effect is one of severe disruption to the balance and equilibrium systems in the brain. If you tried to walk before the spinning sensation stopped, you would find that you could only stagger, as if inebriated. However, through intensive training, it is possible to develop the brain's capacity for accepting a high degree of disorientation. This is evidenced by the ability of ice skaters to perform very rapid and prolonged spinning movements. Such ability involves developing not only the balance parts of the brain, but also overcoming low level reflexive action that normally comes into play when the body's usual relationship to the environment is threatened.

This reflexive action can be very powerful, so much so that it can over-ride the control of the cortex. Take for instance the reaction of most people when they ride a roller-coaster at an amusement park. Before climbing into the carriage, the cortex is able to rationalize the situation and tell you that it is perfectly safe. As terrifying as it may look, there is no reason to be afraid – after all, how often do you hear about someone being killed on a roller-coaster?

But once you start the ride, it is a different story altogether. As you approach the top of the first rise, the cortex immediately loses control. The lower brain areas interpret the situation as being a life-threatening one – that you are going to go crashing down the other side. In the instant of time available, the cortex has no chance to reassure the lower brain area that it really is quite safe. Instead, the life-preserving reflexes of the lower brain go into immediate action – you grip the bar so tightly that your knuckles turn white, your arms go rigid, your eyes nearly pop out of their sockets, and your face turns as white as a ghost.

What happens next depends to a great degree on your sex. If you are female, you will probably scream; if you are male, you probably won't. It seems that it is socially acceptable – in fact, expected – for females to scream on a roller-coaster. Some males like to use this as an example of the 'weaker sex' argument. But don't believe for one moment any male who tells you that he never gets scared on a

roller-coaster. Males usually react in the same way as do females –
the only difference is that society dictates that it is not in keeping
with their masculine image to scream, so they do all they can to
keep their mouths closed. But as macho as they may be, they cannot
do anything about being scared, for this is the natural response of
the lower brain areas.

The responsibility of the lower brain in such situations is to prepare the body in case of an emergency. You cannot control reactions like fear, nor should you want to. They are there for a very
special purpose – as you would soon discover in a real-life
crisis.

The same type of reaction would happen if you were walking
home late one night down a dark street and someone suddenly came
up from behind and grabbed you. Here, almost everybody would
admit that it is acceptable to scream. Strange as it may seem, this
usually is not the first thing that happens. The cortex may think that
the best reaction is to scream for help, but the lower brain, now in
control, has more important things to do first. In order to prepare
the body for the emergency, adrenalin is pumped into the system,
every muscle goes tense, and the eyes open wide. Then, and only
then, will you be able to scream out. The reflex actions, directed by
the lower brain, have taken priority.

When a little baby is being swung around, these vital reflexes are
being activated, providing stimulation to an essential part of the
brain, and helping to ensure the development of balance and equilibrium. Being thrown and spun around as a baby, then rolling and
spinning yourself as a child, is obviously an important part of development.

However, this is something that many brain injured children
often miss out on, especially if they have severe problems. Sometimes, health or physical disabilities may prevent such activities
being carried out, but often it is due to the general impression that
these children are 'fragile' and need special handling. However,
suitable spatial activities *can* be found for even the most severe
cases.

There are many studies that have demonstrated the importance
of spatial stimulation. All of these point to the fact that children not
exposed to these movements could be adversely affected, and not
just in the balance and vital reflex functions. Young[1] found that rats
stimulated by rapid rotation in a cage, for just three minutes on the

second to fifth days after birth, were superior to rats not exposed to this movement, when tested in a maze one month later. He also found that the harmful effects of drugs given to the mother rat during pregnancy were partially reduced in their effect on the newborns, if these young rats were given early spatial stimulation. Levine[2], a psychologist in the U.S.A., consistently found that rats developed better perceptually and emotionally, if they were physically handled in infancy – a process that would inevitably involve some spatial stimulation.

Here is another example of deprivation caused by brain injury. Already we have seen that brain injured children usually do not spend very much time on the floor, and they miss out on different types of environmental sensory stimulation. Now it can be seen that they also do not get as many balance and spatial activities as normal children usually receive. In view of this, spatial activities should comprise an important part of the treatment program for nearly all types of brain injured children.

Such an approach is advocated by many professionals in the field. For example, Jean Ayers[3] states that:

Vestibular (spatial) stimulation is one of the most powerful tools available for therapeutic use in the remediation of sensory integrative dysfunction.

She goes on to say:

If a child's brain appears to have been insufficiently responsive to vestibular stimuli during his life, therapy probably should provide a bombardment of stimulation through the many different vestibular receptors.'

The type of spatial stimulation given to each child depends on the nature and severity of his problem. If the child has no major difficulties with balance, spatial activities such as rolling, swinging by the arms and legs, and upside-down swinging may be incorporated into the overall stimulation program. If the child does have a balance problem, the use of these activities would need to be increased, and others introduced.

Sometimes, people react adversely to the sight of a brain injured child being rolled along the floor or swung upside down, even though the child more than likely is enjoying himself. They think it is cruel to subject the child to such seemingly harsh treatment. But what about the normal child who just loves to be swung by his ankles, so much so that when you start playing this game with him, he never wants to stop? Since some people feel sorry for a brain injured child, they view these otherwise fun-giving activities as being unfair and unnecessary.

Great care needs to be taken to ensure that any spatial activity being used is safe for the child. With adequate care, there is no reason why such important activities cannot be successfully performed. Besides, for most brain injured children, these spatial activities are usually the favourite part of their treatment program!

A final word to the fathers reading this book: yes, men *do* have instincts – well, at least one! So next time you feel that uncontrollable urge to go and pick up your child and swing him around, *do it*, it's good for him. Even if you don't feel this desire, do it anyway, because your child, whether brain injured or normal, needs it.

Section V
Treating the Whole Child

CHAPTER TWENTY-TWO

No More Pigeon Holes

SINCE so many different labels are used to describe the various symptoms of brain injury, it is no wonder that parents of brain injured children often go from doctor to doctor, and therapist to therapist, in an attempt to find an answer to their child's many problems. But as established earlier, these problems are not all that different from each other – they all stem from the one cause, the injury to the brain.

A brain injured child may be seen by a physiotherapist for his mobility problems, a speech therapist for his lack of speech, an orthopaedist for his orthopaedic problems, an occupational therapist for his feeding difficulties, and a psychiatrist for his emotional immaturity. All of these professionals have something to contribute to the child's welfare and they may offer some valuable assistance, but there is a danger in a multi-disciplined approach in that each specialist will only look at the one aspect of the child's problem that directly concerns him or her. By placing the child into a pigeon hole that says 'speech problem' or 'feeding problem', the inter-relationship that does exist between the various problems may be overlooked.

As we mentioned in Chapter 15, the brain works as a whole – the various parts do not work in complete isolation from each other. Therefore, the treatment of a particular problem may involve working with a seemingly unrelated area. A speech therapist, if only looking at the direct manifestations of the speech problem, may overlook the potential value of using the lower movement stages to help develop the speech pathway. A physiotherapist, in dealing with an immobile child, may utilize all the proper treatment techniques designed to activate the movement part of the brain, but if the child has a severe tactile problem that is not recognized, no significant progress can be made unless the tactile deficiency is directly treated.

Sometimes, this pigeon holing can result in rather unfortunate situations. Take, for instance, the case of one patient who was brain injured as a result of meningitis contracted when she was a baby, resulting in her being blind and unable to walk. When she was almost three, her parents went along to the local blind school hoping that they would get some help in trying to develop their child's vision. However, they were told that the blind school was unable to do anything at that time because of her mobility problem. It was suggested that instead the parents take their child to the local spastic centre. So, off they went – only to be told that the spastic centre couldn't help because of the child's visual problem. It was then suggested that they go and see the people at the blind school . . .

These poor parents, and their child, were left in limbo because of the 'other problem'. If only someone had stopped for a moment and said: 'This child cannot move or see because of her brain injury, so if we try and treat the brain, both of these problems may be improved'.

This kind of approach makes a lot of sense. If the therapists and doctors looked at the child's various problems as being manifestations of the brain injury, thus recognizing the common bond between the problems, a more comprehensive treatment program would be developed. Each problem would still need special treatment, but this would be closely coordinated within the whole treatment program, with the various techniques reinforcing one another.

Such a system should help avoid another pitfall of pigeon-holing brain injured children – concentrating on the child's major problems at the exclusion of other seemingly insignificant disabilities. Just because a brain injured child cannot walk or talk, does not mean that his intellect cannot be developed, or that he cannot be taught to read. But, if the treatment is directed only towards his lack of speech or movement, these other important areas may be overlooked. Also, just because a child is severely brain injured does not mean that what he eats and drinks is less vitally important, or that it is unnecessary to investigate possible allergies to foods and environmental chemicals.

Often, in these situations the attitude is: why concern the parents further, for they already have more than enough to worry about. It is often thought that the child's major problems are so overwhelming that it would not be possible or worthwhile to work on these other areas. But, every attempt should be made to enhance all aspects of the child's development. Even if he never managed to walk or talk, wouldn't it be good if he could learn to read and understand? Think how this would enhance his life.

Pigeons belong in pigeon holes – not children. To ensure a wholistic approach, the symptoms of brain injury should be classified as just that – *'Brain Injury'*.

All aspects of treatment important to the overall development of the child, not only those relevant to the child's major problems, belong in an even bigger category that says: *'The Whole Child'*. The *whole* child has to be looked at, and the *whole* child has to be treated. The next few chapters will look at aspects of this wholistic approach that are often neglected when treating brain injured children.

CHAPTER TWENTY-THREE

Learning to Read

W HEN discussing the topic of teaching brain injured children to read, perhaps the biggest difficulty lies in overcoming the many misconceptions and biases that seem to exist in this area. To make matters worse, we are not only advocating that school-aged brain injured children can and should be taught to read, but that this in fact can be done with these children when they are much younger – even as young as one, two and three.

As well as the old argument of whether or not it is necessary or even possible to teach a seven-year-old brain injured child to read, opposition of another sort arises. Some people do not believe it is possible to teach a normal two-year-old to read, let alone a brain injured child of that age. Even though there is now ample evidence to show that normal children can be taught many intellectual skills, including reading, at an early age, it is to be expected that some people will remain sceptical of this previously unrecognized early ability. It follows that they would be even more doubting that this precocious ability exists in brain injured children.

We would like to present a new approach to reading, an approach that may well challenge your current ideas on this subject. You may find yourself rejecting or resisting this new concept even before you have had a chance to assess it rationally, for old ideas die hard. To enable us to present our case adequately, we ask that for the moment you try and put out of your mind the ideas that you may already have about teaching children to read. In fact, try and imagine that you have no knowledge about how and when children learn to read.

Before we begin, it needs to be said that this chapter is as much about normal children as it is about those who are brain injured. The principles involved in teaching both groups to read are almost identical. A few special rules apply to some brain injured children, and these will be explained later.

In Chapter 10, you may have noticed that on the Sandler-Brown Developmental Profile, the ability to read several words was credited to eighteen- to twenty-four-month-old children. When you first saw this, you may have thought it was a printing error; it wasn't, for children of this age have the neurological ability to learn to read, that is, the brain has developed all the necessary tools required for reading to take place. The reason why not many two-year-olds are reading is not because they are unable to at this age, but simply because they have not yet been taught. If they are shown how, most two-year-olds *can* learn to read.

The problem is that most adults underestimate the ability and intelligence of young children. They cannot imagine that a child so little can learn to do something as complicated as reading. The truth is that most two- and three-year-olds have begun to learn to read anyway, despite the fact that nobody has directly taught them.

Most parents will have experienced this situation. You are driving in the car, and you pass the hamburger store with its sign so prominently displayed. Suddenly, your two-year-old yells out that he wants a hamburger, even though he may never have had one in his life. Have you ever stopped to wonder just how he knew which shop sold hamburgers? No one mentioned the word as you drove past, so how did he know? It is called the power of television advertising. By unwittingly being exposed to the hamburger store's intensive advertising campaign, he has learnt to associate the sign above the store with a delicious looking hamburger. He has in fact learnt to make the abstract connection between a sign, or a symbol, and the real object. Although he is responding to a symbol rather than a word, he is using the same process that is involved in learning how to read.

Just how does reading develop? Some people think of it as an educational process, something that children are taught to do when they go to school or preschool. However, we look at reading as being a *neurological* function that can develop as soon as the brain reaches a suitable level of maturity. It serves as another pathway to the brain, by which the brain receives information from the environment.

The neurological process involved in learning to read is very similar to that utilized in the development of understanding. The information is received by the eyes rather than the ears, and different areas of the brain are involved, but the basic process is the same. To understand this, let's look at the way a baby learns to comprehend the spoken word.

Most parents will talk to their baby even when he is tiny and unable to understand. They do not wait until he is nine- to twelve-months-old, the age when a baby should begin to comprehend speech, before they start talking to him. Speech is part of the natural bonding relationship between parent and baby. Parents realize they have to talk to their child so that he will eventually know what they are saying – if he never hears any words, he will never understand.

Infants identify sounds and appreciate what they mean before they comprehend words. For instance, a nine-month-old may not know the word 'bath', but as soon as he hears the sound of running water coming from the bathroom he knows what is coming next. The auditory pathway is not yet mature enough to decipher words, but it can identify specific sounds.

As the understanding of words begins to develop, the infant does not hear the words as we do. He does not hear 'mummy' as 'mummee', but rather hears a sound which is different from all the other sounds surrounding him. Every time he hears 'mum-mee', it's connected to that nice warm person who feeds and looks after him most of the time. Every time he hears the sound for 'daddy' it is associated with that person who has a gruff voice and whiskers on his face.

He hears sounds over and over again that are specific to a particular object or person, and the connection between the two is eventually made. There is nothing significant about the particular sound of a word that makes it easy for him to understand. For example, if the mother called herself a cat, the child would grow up addressing his mother as 'cat'. Rather, it is simply the constant repetition and association that enables the child to connect sounds and objects together. As his auditory pathway becomes more mature, he begins to hear the word 'mummy' as we do. Now he can hear words, instead of just word-like sounds.

The same kind of process takes place when a child first learns to read. Initially he doesn't see the word as we do, but rather as a strange configuration of lines and shapes that is different from other configurations that he may have been shown. Instead of *'Mummy'*, he sees lines and shapes that are different from those in the word *'Daddy'*. Each time he sees those particular lines and shapes, they are associated with a certain sound and object, and he eventually makes the connection. As well, he eventually begins to see the word *'Mummy'* as we do.

This is the same process which adults use when they are in a foreign country and cannot read the native language. There are two words that have to be learnt very quickly so as to prevent any embarrassing situations – 'men' and 'women'. Imagine walking into what you thought was the men's room, only to discover that your reading ability was not quite as good as you hoped it was! These days, little stick figures on the doors avoid any embarrassing moments. But, imagine that you are in a remote part of Greece where tourists never go. Seeing that all the locals are literate, they have no reason to use diagrams as well as words. To make matters worse, the Greek alphabet is completely different to your own, so there is no way that you can guess. Thus, there are two words that you will very quickly memorize:

$$ANΔPΩN = \text{MEN}$$

$$ΓYNAIKΩN = \text{WOMEN}$$

You are not able to pronounce these words, and you don't even know which letters of the alphabet are being used. But every time you see those strange configurations of lines and shapes, you understand exactly what they mean. If you stay in Greece long enough, you undoubtedly will learn to read other important words in this fashion.

Can such a process be described as 'reading'? After all, you can't even spell or pronounce the words. However, you can achieve what the basic purpose of reading involves – relating a specific meaning to a written word. As far as the Greek language is concerned, it is only the very beginning of this skill, but it is reading. After all, the only thing that reading consists of in the beginning is the memorization of different sets of lines and shapes, at the same time learning what each set represents.

The method by which you would learn to read those important Greek words is the same way that a child learns to read. It is also very similar to the method by which he learns to understand – and by which you would learn to understand other Greek words that you hear rather than see.

If reading is so straightforward, then why aren't more two- and three-year-olds able to read? It is simply a matter of not being taught. Neurologically, at this age they possess all the tools necessary for the function of reading to occur – they are able to identify pictures and recognize detail within pictures, so the visual pathway is suitably developed. In addition, they have an extremely large vocabulary of words that they can understand – so the process similar to that of reading has already been established through the auditory pathway.

Thus, everything is there and waiting, all that is needed is someone to teach them. Thinking back to the example of the two-year-old learning to 'read' the hamburger sign, it seems that television has beaten most parents to the task. However, this initial exposure to the skill of reading does not usually come from the educational shows. These programs are well produced and are quite effective as a teaching medium, but there is something better than this – the advertisements.

Most of you who are parents will have witnessed the following scene: your two-year-old is happily playing in another room while you are watching the television. As soon as his favourite commercail comes on, he drops whatever he is playing with and comes rushing into the living room. He then stands about twenty centimetres from the television, completely engrossed in what is on the screen. As soon as the advertisement is over, he goes back into the other room and resumes his game.

You see, the advertising agencies are very clever, for they know exactly how best to get information into the brain. And not only that, they know how to make sure it stays there – for adults as well as children. It's called frequency, intensity and duration – those three magic words you heard so much about in Chapter 16.

Frequency – we all know how often some of the advertisements are repeated, almost to saturation point. Intensity – most ads are not known for their subtlety. Rather, they use the attention-gaining abilities of colour and sound to their fullest. Duration – not only are they repeated several times each night, but ads never seem to go away. They are screened night after night, day after day.

This is why two-year-olds can recognize the hamburger store. It is also what infuriates adults when they hear a lovely piece of classical music, and immediately think about a brand of cigarettes that used this music for its promotion.

Now, we are not advocating for one moment that you sit your two- and three-year-olds in front of the television and make them watch all of the advertisements. Instead, a lesson should be learnt from the advertising agencies, so that these already proven techniques can be used to teach young children to read.

First of all, just like the ads, the words have to be shown lots and lots of times. When you are teaching a baby to understand, you have to repeat the words over and over again before the message sinks in. Children learn best by repetition, and this is especially true in regard to reading. The words should be shown very briefly. Children have a very short attention span, so they will not sit patiently for very long. Instead, they will be off in one or two minutes, looking for something else to do. Rather than trying to make them sit for longer, the words should be shown for the brief moment their attention is captured. It is much more effective to have very short sessions repeated frequently during the day instead of two or three long periods.

Also, the appropriate intensity needs to be applied. A two-year-old's visual pathway is not mature enough to read small print, so the words need to be clearly printed in lower case letters (with capital used where appropriate), in large, bold lettering – usually five to eight cms high (two to three inches), using a bright-coloured ink (preferably red) on white cardboard. Just as in the advertisement, the words need to be shown in a dramatic fashion so that the child can't help being attracted to what you are presenting. For that moment, you need to become an actor.

You should not expect a child to learn to read in a week or two. After all, when his understanding was developing, it took weeks and months of hearing the same words over and over again before he began to recognize what they meant. Thus, the reading words need to be shown daily, over many months to enable the child to build up a reading vocabulary.

The rate at which new words should be introduced varies with each child. Care should be taken to ensure that you advance according to the child's progress, rather than by what is said in this or any other book. The danger in giving instructions about how to teach a child to read is that it will be done 'by the book' instead of by the child.

Having given this warning, the following is a general outline of how to organize a reading program. Adaptations should be made to suit the individual child. You should begin by choosing the five words which are the most meaningful to your child – these will probably include 'mummy, 'daddy', your child's name, and anything else that appeals to him. If you are the child's mother, when you show the word 'mummy' hold it up and, in a very animated voice say: 'Look Mary, this says mummy, and that's me!' Or, if you show the word 'daddy', hold it up and tell her what it says, then either point to daddy, if he is around, or show her a photograph of him – this is best put on the reverse side of the card. That is all you have to do – it really is as simple as that.

You should use the same five words for the first two weeks, showing them many, many times each day for very brief periods. At the end of the two weeks, you may feel the need to test your child to see if he knows any of the five words that you have been showing him. However, at this stage it would be best if you didn't. Your desire to check his progress is probably based on a vague feeling of scepticism or amazement that your child can really be learning something that you have always thought to be very difficult. But think about when you were teaching your child to understand – you didn't feel the need to constantly test him. You didn't say: 'Hi Johnny, I'm your mummy – who *am* I?' You had faith that as long as you put all the right information in, he would eventually understand. So, why not adopt the same approach with reading? In these early stages, have faith that it is going to work, and just show him the words – you can worry about testing later on.

At the end of the first two weeks, you should begin introducing new words. Initially, it is best to teach a new word every two days. During these two days, you should continue showing the old words, but concentrate mostly on the new one. At the same time, you should reinforce the new word in other ways. For instance, if you introduce the word 'hand', you should continually talk about his hand, so that he is not only seeing the word, he is also hearing it and being taught what it means. For a very young child, this will help his understanding as much as it will develop his reading.

After six to eight weeks, you can begin testing your child if you so desire, but at this point it is still not really necessary. If you do want to test him, it is very simple – all you do is hold up two words, and ask him to choose the word that you are saying. He can point to the word, look at it, or pick it up – whatever the child wants to do. If he gets it right, you may think that he is guessing, but if he chooses the correct word seven or eight times out of ten, you can assume that he knows these words. If he does get them right, you must immediately let him know how clever you think he is. If he discovers that reading is a great way of getting lots of love and attention, he should learn to like it very quickly. Even if your child enjoys being tested, it should not be done very often, and there certainly should be no stress involved.

If your child gets most of the words right when you test him, or if you just feel that he is going well and is enjoying his reading, you can start to show him a new word every day. At this point, you don't need to show all of the old words each day, just five or six different ones daily should be enough. Instead, you should concentrate mostly on the new word, reinforcing it in as many ways as possible. If you are teaching words that describe things around the house, it is a good idea to make another copy of the word and attach it to the real object – 'stove' should be prominently displayed on the stove, so that every time he is in the kitchen, he can associate the word to the real object.

At some point, you may think that your child is not grasping some of the new words, or he is losing interest in the whole process. You may need to slow down the rate of introducing new words, or you may need to spend more time reviewing the old words. Again, adjustments have to be made according to the individual child.

You can teach any words that you wish, but in the beginning it is best to use ones that he can relate to, such as body parts and household objects. Always give a clear explanation of the word at a level that your child would understand, and where possible, put a big and attractive picture on the back of the card, so he can see what the real object looks like.

A mistake that is often made is to teach a child simple, short words, in the belief that these are the easiest words to learn. However, it is the other way around. 'Cat', 'sat' and 'mat' are very similar, as are 'hair' and 'chair', and someone just learning to read could be easily confused by these words. On the other hand, 'television' and 'refrigerator' look and sound very different. Thus, it is these long words that children find easiest to read, and they also love to hear you say these words, for they sound funny to them.

Perhaps the most common mistake made when teaching children to read is to introduce new words too slowly. This often results in the child becoming bored, as he continues to see words that he already knows. Young children are desperate for *new* information, and are not usually satisfied by things they already know. Thus, he may rapidly lose interest with the same old reading words, and he will look away or switch off whenever the words are brought out. Unfortunately, his actions are often misinterpreted, for it is thought that his lack of attention is a sign that he is unable to learn. Therefore, his parents keep on showing him the words he already knows and is completely bored with, and everyone concerned becomes frustrated and fed up with the whole thing.

Usuully such a situation occurs for three reasons:

● The intelligence of young children is underestimated.

● It is assumed that you have to proceed very slowly if such a young child is to learn such a supposedly complicated task.

● It is thought that a child has to learn almost all the words he is shown, before he sees any new words.

This third point is contrary to the established principles of learning. Adults only learn a fraction of what they are taught – common estimates are that only about 30 per cent of all information presented is retained. *You* don't learn everything you are taught, so why should you expect this of your child? There may be some words that he has trouble with, or simply doesn't like, but there is no point in slowing down the whole process because of these few words. Obviously, he needs to know most of the words (around 70 per cent), but not all of them. Referring back to the development of understanding, you don't make sure a child understands a particular word before you introduce another one – you expose him to lots of words at the one time, knowing that he will eventually understand most of them.

There is a choice between two basic approaches that can be used to teach a child to read. You can take the 'slow and steady' method, by which a very cautious attitude is adopted. Over a nine month period, you can show your child a total of fifty words, advancing to a new word only when you think he knows the previous one. At the end of this period you test him, and discover that he has done extremely well, for he can read forty-five of the fifty words – a 90 per cent success rate. However, there is an inherent danger in such an approach. There is a good chance that your child may become so bored with this slow pace that he rapidly loses interest in anything remotely connected to reading. If you continue for too much longer in this fashion, he may switch off altogether.

The alternative method would be to show lots and lots of words, assuming that he will learn a good proportion of these, but without expecting him to learn every single one. Over a nine month period, you may show as many as 200 words. However, a test at the end of this time may show that the child knows only 50 per cent of the words. This seems a dismal result compared to the 90 per cent success rate of the other method. But, look again, for the child has learnt 100 words – more than twice the number of the slow and steady approach. As well as being far superior in terms of the total number of words learnt, this method also helps to prevent boredom. With so many new words to see, the child should find it immensely enjoyable.

As you probably will have guessed, this second method is the one that we suggest for most children. But, as we said earlier, the method that is best suited to each individual child is the one that should be adopted, and the approach should be a flexible one, based on how the child is responding.

You may have been wondering why we haven't made any special reference so far to teaching brain injured children how to read. Well, until now it simply has not been necessary, because the principles we have been discussing apply equally to brain injured and normal children. However, there are certain exceptions that obviously require a different approach. If a child has a severe understanding or visual problem that prevents the information from being received by the brain, then the therapy program would initially have to concentrate on these areas. Once these basic functions were improved, a reading program could be introduced.

In the case of a child with a less severe visual or understanding problem, a modified reading program should be introduced, as apart from hopefully teaching the child to read, such a process should also help to develop the visual and auditory pathways. For this child, the words should be written in bigger, bolder letters, they should be shown more often, with the new words being introduced at a slower rate. Special emphasis should also be placed on teaching the understanding of each word.

Special allowances often need to be made when testing a brain injured child. Since he may not be able to point to or say the correct word, a means of communication needs to be established by which he can show the required word. He may be able to turn his head, or even just look with his eyes – this is all that is needed. Even if the child's physical disabilities prevent any form of communication, this is *not* a reason for ignoring the reading program. Just because he cannot show you the correct word does not mean that he is unable to read. Many children, despite their severe physical problems, have become very proficient readers – so an attempt should be made to try and develop this skill in such cases.

In most instances, little importance should be placed on whether or not the child can say the words that he is reading. There is no direct relationship between the ability to say and read a word, for they are two different functions of the brain. This is especially the case with a child who has a speech problem. If you try and assess this child's reading by his oral response to the words, you are confusing his reading ability with his speech disability. Many such children are held back in their reading development because of this misunderstanding.

If your child is learning to read and is making good progress, you are bound to come across at least one sceptic who refuses to accept that a child, not yet out of nappies, could possibly be reading. These people will probably tell you that your child has just memorized the words. If this ever happens to you, simply turn around to them and say: 'I know, isn't that wonderful?' What else is the beginning of reading other than memorizing words? How can a child learn to read if he doesn't memorize?

If they still have their doubts, they will then probably want to know what is the point of teaching such a young child to read. After all, two-year-olds are meant to be content with toys and television, aren't they?

Well, it all depends on the way that you look at reading. If, like us, you consider it to be a basic neurological function, similar to understanding, then you would probably agree that it should be developed while the child is young and anxious to learn. Since the brain is still in a dynamic state of growth and is readily accepting information from the environment, it is much easier to teach a two-year-old than, say, a six-year-old. A two-year-old's brain is like a piece of blotting paper, waiting to soak up all the information that it is given, so why not take advantage of this?

As well, reading is another form of environmental stimulation that will help to develop the brain. It is an additional means by which the brain can learn from the environment.

Apart from this, most children who are taught to read simply love it. They think of it as being just another fun toy to play with. It is fun for the parents too. It is a tremendously rewarding experience to watch your child's eyes light up as you show him his favourite word. At the same time, you know that you are developing what is going to become an important life-time skill.

Above all else, teaching young children to read, be they brain injured or normal, is usually very easy. Thus, learning to read is simple, it is fun, and it is productive.

CHAPTER TWENTY-FOUR

The Slow Learner

IF, AS the last chapter explains, reading is so simple that even two-year-olds can do it, why is it that in almost every classroom in almost every school there is at least one child who has a reading and learning problem? Teaching the good students to read has never been a problem for educators. In fact, these children seem to learn to read regardless of the method used to teach them, and without any apparent effort. Often, they appear to virtually teach themselves. But there is always the child who falls further and further behind his classmates.

Before the days of compulsory education, a slow learning child was all but unheard of. In those days the only children who went to school were those who had rich parents. The others stayed at home or worked in the factories. If a rich child had difficulties with learning, and if the teacher was unable to rectify the problem, the solution was simple – the child was taken away from school, an action which usually ended his formal education.

As soon as laws were introduced enabling all children to receive a formal education, the difficulties involved in teaching slow learners were discovered. Since these children now had to stay at school, the teachers were faced with the problem of devising suitable ways to get the message through. Some children were taught by the look-say method, whereby the whole word was shown and repeated out loud. Others were taught by phonetics, a method which involved breaking the word up into its phonetic components. However, the look-say and phonetic schools still had about the same number of children with learning problems, despite the different techniques.

Various theories were advanced in an attempt to explain why some children were slow learners. The first that was presented is perhaps best described as the stupid Johnny theory. Johnny couldn't learn to read simply because 'he wasn't clever enough'.

But soon it was discovered that Johnny, even though he had problems learning to read, was very good at mathematics, or was quite artistic. It did not make sense, for how could he be good in these other areas if he was not very bright? In fact, many children who have reading difficulties can function very well in skills that do not involve reading, and it is now widely accepted that a reading problem does not necessarily reflect a lack of intelligence. Thus, the stupid Johnny theory was quickly discarded.

Next, the stupid parent theory was introduced into the argument. Johnny couldn't read very well because his parents were not very intelligent, and they had done little to educate him before he went to school. But, it was soon discovered that these supposedly dull parents had raised their two other children very well, with both of these children being among the best readers in their classes. How was it that although the parents weren't bright enough to help Johnny, they had done all the right things with their other children. Needless to say, the stupid parent theory was also quickly dismissed.

The next person to be blamed was the teacher, and the stupid teacher theory was used to explain away all the problems that children were having in school. The teacher was supposedly unable to get the message across to the children, and as a result they were unable to learn the basic skills involved with reading. But how was it that in a class of thirty children, only two or three of them had problems with their reading? If the teacher was not doing his or her job properly, the majority of children should have been having difficulties. The stupid teacher argument lasted about as long as the two other theories.

Psychologists then entered into the argument, announcing that they had discovered that most slow learning children had psychological problems. Therefore, their reading difficulties were in some way related to their poor self-image, or whatever other psychological abnormality was present. Lots of slow learners then began having psychological treatment, but usually all that happened was that they became well adjusted children who still had learning problems. Being a slow learner is enough to give anyone a psychological problem, especially in the competitive world of today where everybody has to be a winner. In other words, the psychological problem was a result of being a slow learner, not the other way around. Some children were helped by the psychological treatment they received, but as a general historical statement, this approach to the problem failed to achieve the desired results.

There was a common denominator in most of the arguments that were being presented to explain why some children could not keep up with their peers, for it was usually referred to as an *educational* problem. Since the symptoms were most obvious in the classroom, it was thought the answer to the problem lay somewhere within the confines of the education discipline. But if this was the case, somewhere along the way appropriate educational treatment should have solved or significantly improved the problems of the slow learner.

However, time and time again, we have seen slow learning children who have received a first-class education. They have been to the best schools, have had the best teachers, yet they still have difficulties in reading and learning. They may have made progress, but their improvement was not significant enough to enable them to perform as well as their peers. Some children have received a lot of help from their teachers, and from various teaching methods, but there are others who continue to make poor progress despite all the efforts that are made to improve the situation. In these situations the teachers and the parents feel they are hitting their heads up against a brick wall, for whatever they try fails to get through to the child. What else could be preventing the child from learning as easily as most other children?

In a radical departure from the general consensus of opinion of the time, a new way of looking at learning problems was presented in the 1950s. Instead of thinking in terms of educational reasons to explain why some children were having trouble keeping up at school, it was suggested that perhaps some of the problems were neurologically based.

In effect, this argument was reverting back to the stupid Johnny theory – although no longer in any way implying that the problem lay in Johnny's lack of intelligence, but pointing to the fact that the problem was within Johnny, and had little to do with which school he attended, how good his teacher was, or what particular teaching methods were employed.

The argument was really quite simple. It was not that Johnny wasn't intelligent enough to read, it was just that his brain was unable to correctly carry out the many complex steps involved in reading. In other words, it was suggested that any interference or hindrance to normal neurological function would adversely affect the reading and learning ability of a child.

Initially, this proposal was met with great scepticism by educators, psychologists and others working in the field. In retrospect, this was a strange reaction. On the one hand, these professionals recognized the necessity of having a properly functioning neurological system for the normal development of all learning. But, on the other hand, they seemed to overlook the obvious fact that if the neurological system was malfunctioning, in all likelihood the learning process would be adversely affected, no matter how slight the malfunction may be.

One of the biggest stumbling blocks to this new theory being accepted was that these slow learning children did not appear to be brain injured in any way. They could walk, talk, run and play, so how on earth could it be suggested that they were brain injured? However, the proponents of this new theory believed it was simply a matter of degree, for being brain injured did not necessarily mean that any obvious symptoms would be detected on superficial examination. If severe brain injury had occurred, then certainly the child's basic functions would be seriously affected. But if the injury was very mild, the effects of the brain's performance may only show up later in life when the brain was required to perform very sophisticated tasks, such as learning to read and write. If a brain malfunction was responsible for the learning problems that the child had, it was thought that the child had suffered only 'minimal brain injury'. Or in some cases it was suggested that the child may not have suffered any injury to the brain at all: instead something had gone wrong during development that caused the brain to be disorganized – a condition referred to as 'neurological disorganization'. Here the brain was likened to a complex electrical circuit board, where every wire had to be in its correct place, making the right connections with the other wires. If the circuit board consisted of ten thousand wires and only one was out of place, then some kind of breakdown may occur. This is especially critical in the human brain where millions and millions of working parts are involved.

With children who had suffered minimal brain injury, it was thought that some minor problem may have occurred during the pregnancy or around the time of birth that affected a seemingly insignificant number of brain cells. The child may have appeared to have developed normally, although when they look back, parents of such children often recall being concerned that their child seemed to be progressing more slowly than normal, or that he was more clumsy than his older brothers and sisters were at his age. The neurologically disorganized children usually were born without complications after uneventful pregnancies; however, for one reason or another, they often did not go through all the developmental stages as other children did. They may not have crawled on their tummy or may have done so only for a short time, or they may not have crawled on their hands and knees, choosing instead to get up and walk early. Or, they may have been very passive, being quite content to just lie or sit for most of the day. In some cases they may have been put in devices such as a walker that limited their time spent moving around on the floor.

Having got this far in this book, and having learnt how the brain grows, develops and performs, this concept of a possible neurological involvement in reading and learning problems probably makes sense to you. This was not the case thirty years ago, and indeed the battle raged for many years after that. Today, these ideas are much more readily accepted, and there are many schools and therapy centres working with slow learning children that include neurologically-based treatment techniques in their therapy programs.

It does make sense that a child could be having learning problems because of some minor dysfunction in the brain. Indeed, our experience in working with children suffering from these kinds of problems has given further credence to this theory. For instance, it has been fascinating to observe how often you find that a slow learning child, who was thought to have developed normally, in fact did not crawl on his tummy, or only crawled on his hands and knees for a very short time, or was a very passive baby who hardly did anything until he got up to walk. In at least 70 per cent of the slow learning children we have seen there has been some part of their development that has been different from the accepted norms, either by completely missing stages or doing them for a very short time. This may be pure coincidence and completely unrelated to the learning problems of the children, but viewed in conjunction with the neurological theory, it's of more than passing interest.

There are other signs common in slow learning children that indicate possible neurological involvement. Many of these children are clumsy and poorly coordinated. They have difficulty learning new physical skills, and it takes a great deal of practice and perseverance for any skill to be mastered. They often have poor spatial awareness, and find it difficult to differentiate their right foot from the left. They can become confused when following directions that have a spatial content, such as 'get the ball off the top of the bookcase and put it behind the door on the right'. They may be hyperactive and have short attention spans, or have drastic mood or behavioural changes for no apparent reason. Some slow learners may suffer from any of these problems in conjunction with their learning problems, some may have just one or two, others may have none at all. However, more often than not these children have at least two or three of these associated problems. Viewed in isolation, these problems do not necessarily indicate some form of neurological dysfunction, as they could be the result of other causes. But if they occur together with learning problems, then it may indicate that both these associated problems and the actual learning disorder have some neurological basis.

If a slow learning child has suffered a minimal brain injury or has become neurologically disorganized, then what of treatment? First it must be realized that not all children who have learning problems are that way because of a dysfunction in their brain, as the cause could be something completely unrelated to the neurological system. Or the brain dysfunction could be only part of the reason why the child is having problems at school. Secondly, neurological treatment on its own will not solve the problem completely, for there are other treatment modalities that must be considered. Appropriate educational techniques have to be employed, motor-perceptual activities included to help improve hand-eye and overall coordination, visual exercises incorporated if a specific visual problem exists. In other words, a comprehensive approach needs to be adopted so that the child's problems can be attacked from *every* conceivable and appropriate angle.

Where there is an indication that there may be neurological involvement in the learning problem, appropriate neurological techniques should be incorporated into the treatment program. It is often difficult to prove a direct neurological dysfunction. It will not show up when investigative techniques such as a CAT scan or an EEG machine are used, and there may be nothing in the history of the pregnancy and birth that would indicate that the brain has been injured. But if some of the associated problems mentioned earlier are present, or if the child's development history did not conform to normal, then it would be wise to utilize neurological techniques as part of the treatment offered. The child could only benefit from this action as these techniques are virtually harmless.

The neurological approach to the treatment of learning problems is based on the principle that the correct foundations have to be laid in the brain for future development to build on. Proper development at the early stages of brain growth will help ensure the integrity of the subsequent higher and more sophisticated levels of the brain. It is exactly the same principle that is involved in building a house. Let's imagine that when you decided to build a house, your only concern was to make sure it was the best looking home in the neighbourhood. You wanted people to drive by and think to themselves: 'What a beautiful house, those people must be rich'. Seeing that these people were only going to notice what was built above the ground, you decided not to waste any money on foundations. After all, no one would ever ask if they could look at the what was below the ground. With all the money that you saved, you could make the house look even fancier.

So, you instruct your builder not to worry about putting foundations in and to go ahead and build the house directly on top of the ground. No builder would agree to such a proposal, but for the sake of the argument let's suppose that your builder does. When he has finished his work, you realize that your dream has come true, for your house is in a class of its own. Every second car slows down to enable the occupants to have a look, and you can almost see them turn green with envy. Strange values, but you have got exactly what you wanted.

However, you soon begin to question the wisdom of your decision not to put foundations in. Within six months you notice small cracks appearing in some of the walls, and as time goes by these cracks grow bigger and become more numerous. On this occasion you cannot blame the builder, for your decision to do away with the foundations is directly responsible for the cracks appearing. As the natural movement and erosion of the ground upon which the house is built occurs, the house has no choice but to move too. But, houses are designed to remain stationary, so any movement will eventually result in cracks appearing in the walls. This is the simple reason why money has to be spent to put in suitable foundations.

As the cracks continue to worsen, you have the choice of two actions whereby you may remedy the problem. You can take the easiest and cheapest way – and based on your record so far, this is almost certainly what you will do. This simply involves patching up the holes with plaster and then painting over them. Initially it would seem that this course of action has been effective, for you can no longer notice where the cracks were. But, this improvement will be only temporary, and the cracks will all reopen and continue to develop in new places. The reason is quite simple – the problem is not in the walls for there is nothing wrong with the structure of the wall itself. By patching up the cracks you are simply treating the symptoms of the problem.

Your other choice is to tackle the cause of the problem. Like it or not, the only way you can do this is to jack the house up, put the foundations in, and then lower the house down. A very expensive procedure, but the only way that you can save your house. Even if you had employed the best builder and the best architect, and used only the finest building materials, there is no way you could have avoided those cracks appearing without the house being on proper foundations. Furthermore, the cracks in the walls would be just the start of your worries. In the end the house will fall down if the movement becomes severe. In other words a house is only as good as the foundations it is built on.

This is also true of the human brain. The higher cortical levels, the parts of the brain responsible for our most sophisticated intellectual abilities, do not function independently of the lower brain areas. Indeed, if the lower areas are not developed correctly or completely, there can be drastic consequences in the higher levels. Chapter 12 in this book stated that 'you have to walk before you can run', and this is true for the development of all the various learning skills as it is for the development of any other brain function. Therefore, if a child did not crawl on his tummy or on hands and knees, or did these movements for just a short time, or in a poorly coordinated fashion, then it may have an effect upon his later learning. Even if a child did go through these developmental stages at the times he was supposed to do so and seemed to spend a lot of time moving in these ways, he may not have done enough to ensure that his brain had completed its development. There is no average requirement, no predetermined amount of early developmental activities needed to ensure correct brain growth, and each person has different levels of input and output that their brain requires to develop normally.

This does not mean to say that every child who does not achieve all the normal milestones will develop a learning problem. Nor does it follow that every person who has a minimal brain injury or neurological disorganization will become a slow learner. There are many children who skip stages who are absolutely normal in every way, and there are others who despite apparent mild injury to the brain do not show any outward effects. These cases serve to illustrate just how amazingly adaptable the human brain is, how it can compensate when things go slightly wrong or not according to schedule.

However, there are some children who are susceptible to any variation from the normal pathway of development. These children are at risk if they do not spend adequate time on the floor when they are young, given that being on the floor helps the child to use and explore all the appropriate developmental activities and movements. It is also important to note that those children who suffer mild brain injury are often passive babies who are slow to develop. They sometimes even skip developmental stages, or do some developmental activities and movements for just short periods of time. Thus they are at risk in two ways – firstly because of the brain injury suffered, and secondly because they then develop in a way that can cause neurological disorganization in otherwise normal children. If one doesn't get them, then the other one might.

The neurological part of the treatment program is as simple as the rationale behind it. It involves neuro-developmental activities such as tummy crawling, crawling on hands and knees, rolling, spinning, somersaulting, and coordination and balance activities. The proportion of time spent on each activity, and the total amount of time required each day depends on each child, but it may be as little as one hour a day for a child with minor problems, to several hours a day for a more severely affected child. Many children continue to attend school full time and do their exercises before and after school, or others go to school on a part-time basis so they have time to do a more extensive neurological program.

As mentioned earlier, the neurological treatment is only part of the whole program that should be given to these children. Time needs to be spent on remedial teaching, normal socialization, perceptual-motor activities, and any other specific treatments that the child may require. Other factors need to be considered in this wholistic approach to the slow learner. For instance, diet often plays a vital role in helping these children, especially if the child is also hyperactive. A diet based on the principles outlined in the next chapter should be established and carefully adhered to. Allergies are often a major contributing factor to the problems of the slow learner, and this is further explained in Chapter 26. If a child has a poor self-image or is not motivated to improve himself, then psychological guidance may be of help if it is combined with all the other suggested courses of action.

Educational treatment given in isolation is unlikely to enable the slow learner to reach his greatest potential, for the problem is often more than just educational. Psychological guidance given in isolation is also unlikely to reach this goal, as the problem is often more than just psychological. Neurological treatment given without any attention being paid to other contributing factors will also fail to achieve the ultimate goal, as the problem is often more than just neurological. All these aspects of treatment, along with correct diet, attention to possible allergies, and anything else that is appropriate to the individual child, have to be combined into a wholistic program if the best results are to be obtained.

However, the neurological part of the treatment often holds the key for real success, as the child can only learn as well as his brain will allow him to. If the function of the brain is improved, then all the learning activities that were previously so difficult should gradually become easy, and the child will be much more receptive to what he is taught.

Perhaps the example of Craig best demonstrates the important role neurological treatment plays in helping the slow learner: we first saw Craig when he was fourteen, after he had been attending a very good special school for seven years. Unfortunately, his was a very severe case of dyslexia, and after all that time at a special school all he could read was his own name. Since they had done all they could do to help him without success, his teachers had resigned themselves to the fact that Craig probably would never be able to read. They had stopped a formal education program, and instead they were now trying to teach him living skills. We devised a neuro-developmental program for Craig that involved working two hours a day on the therapy techniques described earlier. He continued to go to school, doing his therapy program before and after school each day.

When Craig returned for reassessment three months later, he walked in with a large bundle of words under his arm. With a big smile on his face, he announced that he could read all of the words he had brought with him – all 200 of them! We proceeded to test him, and much to our amazement we discovered that not only could he identify each of the words, he could also comprehend their meanings. The only thing that Craig was doing now that was different to what he had been doing before was the crawling, rolling and vision work, and all the other activities that were in his therapy program, so it seemed that these neuro-developmental techniques were achieving the desired results. In the eighteen months that Craig carried out the therapy, he improved his reading up to a third grade level, an excellent result, given that normal children usually take three years from the time that they begin school until they reach third grade reading standard.

Although Craig had received a very good education, it wasn't until the proper neurological foundations were laid down that he was able to begin to learn (it is relevant that Craig had never crawled on his tummy or hands and knees when he was a baby). By developing the parts of his brain that now seemed to have been necessary for his learning, he then was able to accept and process the information being presented to him.

Of course it is not always as easy as that, and it does not always work as well, but Craig's story illustrates the importance of using neuro-developmental techniques in the treatment of slow learners when the indications are that it may be of value.

CHAPTER TWENTY-FIVE

Nutrition

PARENTS of brain injured children often feel frustrated because there seems to be so little they can do for their child; they feel deeply sorry for him and desperately want to do something – anything – to make him happy. If they can do nothing else, at least they can try and put a smile on his face.

They soon discover that there is one thing from which most children derive pleasure – food. Their child, despite his other difficulties, still has a good sense of taste with a liking for certain foods. Much to his parents' relief, eating is at least one thing that makes him happy.

Advertisers have also realized that food is a good way of making people 'happy' and it hasn't taken them long to discover the marketing potential of 'happy foods'. This theme features prominently in many of their advertising campaigns. For example, a particular brand of carbonated drink is supposed to make you so happy that you smile – this message is reinforced by the sight of a healthy looking group of teenagers with big smiles on their faces.

There is nothing wrong with using food as a means of bringing enjoyment to the life of a child who misses out on most other pleasures – provided the food is wholesome, nutritious and free of chemical additives such as preservatives, artificial colours and flavours, stabilizers, and emulsifiers. Unfortunately, this is not the case with many of the 'happy foods' marketed today. They may taste good, and your child may certainly enjoy them, but they may have both immediate and long term detrimental effects on his health.

In today's world of high technology, our whole philosophy towards eating has become confused. If the function of eating is looked at from a purely scientific viewpoint, the *only* reason for the consumption of food is to supply the body with the essential nutrients that these foods contain. Without food, we simply cannot survive. It is not just a matter of eating any foods – great care has to be taken to ensure that a proper selection is made. Certain foods are of higher quality than others, and a wide variety needs to be consumed to ensure that a complete range of nutrients is received.

Thus, if eating is approached scientifically, the first consideration that needs to be made when choosing which foods to eat is the nutritive value of each food. In other words, people should be asking: 'Is this food good for me?'

But how many people can honestly say that this is the first thing that comes to mind when they sit down to have breakfast in the morning? If you are like most people, your first consideration is: 'How good will it taste?' You may give some thought to its nutritional quality, but then again you may be so impressed by its delicious taste that you aren't too concerned about whether or not it is good for you.

The 'pleasure factor' of a food has assumed, for most people, a much higher priority than its potential goodness. Such an attitude would be completely acceptable if all the foods that we ate were of high nutritional quality. But in this age of highly refined and processed foods, this is definitely not the case.

Many of the foods that are advertised as tasting nice are of low nutritional value. These so called 'happy foods', the ones that are meant to make you smile, would make you frown if you knew what ingredients they contained, and what effect these substances can have on your body.

However, the food industry is very good at what it does. You have to hand it to them, for they can take a food that is almost completely devoid of essential nutrients, and make it taste delicious! And here is the trap, for not many people – especially children – can resist the temptation of nice-tasting food, even when they know that it is of poor nutritional quality.

Unfortunately most parents are not aware of the consequences of eating such food. Nor are they aware that it is an absolute necessity that their child receives a diet of the highest quality, unless they have done some reading themselves – or have been lucky enough to find a nutritionally orientated health professional. More than likely, parents will have found that their doctor has placed little emphasis on the importance of good nutrition for brain injured children. Apart from some rather vague advice that they only need to give their child a well balanced diet, they probably will not have received any special instructions.

The myth of the 'well balanced diet' continues, with the general belief that in most Western countries the people eat very well. Thus, we have been led to think that all we have to worry about is the taste appeal of the food, since all the needs of the body will be met by this 'well balanced diet' found on the supermarket shelves. Strange as it may seem, such a belief was closer to the truth in the days of our grandparents and great-grandparents.

If we could venture back to those 'good old days', we would see that they were indeed good as far as nutrition was concerned. People ate wholesome foods that were grown in mineral-rich soils, without the need of chemical sprays and fertilizers. These foods were not processed, over-refined, or kept in storage for months. Since the food was fresh and of high quality, it did not need to be artificially coloured, flavoured or preserved. The animals from which they obtained their meat and eggs were raised without chemical additions to their foods, and they lived in a natural habitat. Our grandparents' intake of refined carbohydrates, especially sugar, was considerably less than today. The air they breathed, the water they drank, and the houses they lived in were not contaminated by harmful chemicals and pollutants.

Of course, there have been many positive advances in food technology since those days, and considerable progress has been made in many aspects of the food industry. Through improved farming techniques and increased scientific understanding of all aspects of agriculture, we are now able to eat a much wider variety of foodstuffs. The preparation of foods is more hygienic and thus the risk of infection from consuming contaminated foods has decreased. As a result of extensive research, more stable and productive crops have been produced.

However, much of the modern day food industry is geared to mass production, and it is here that we run into major problems. Foods are prepared and produced in the knowledge that they are not going to be consumed immediately. They may in fact spend many months in a warehouse or even on a supermarket shelf before being purchased and eventually eaten.

Since these foods need to have a relatively long shelf life, they have to be preserved by some means. In a sense, the food industry had to find a way to defy Nature, for she had designed most foods to be eaten soon after picking or killing. If they were not eaten, they would become infected with bacteria and would quickly go rotten. In the search for a suitable method of food preservation, the values of chemical additives and the means of processing and refining foods were discovered. It was learnt that by removing most of the germ and outer layers of wheat and other grains, the refined product took longer to become rancid and therefore its shelf life was extended. It was also realized that by the addition of certain chemicals, some foods could be preserved quite successfully and for long periods of time. With these important discoveries, the preservation of foods became almost universal.

In the 'old days' it was not necessary to extend the life of most food as it was produced and consumed within a small community. Since there was little or no refrigeration, foods were produced in accordance with daily needs and many foods were purchased and eaten on the same day. Instead of weekly trips to the supermarket, regular visits to the corner store were made to buy the day's requirements. There were daily door-to-door deliveries of perishables such as milk and bread and the greengrocer's cart travelled the streets at least twice a week.

Successful food preservation has been of tremendous importance to the food producers and retailers of today. As well, the consumer has been largely protected from deteriorated, rancid and spoiled foods. However, there is a serious flaw in the principle of extending food life. The methods used have been successful in making most foods more stable, but at the same time they have contributed to the decline in the nutritional quality of what we eat.

Take for instance the refining and processing of grain products such as wheat. It works well as a means of preservation, simply because it removes almost all of the biologically active parts of the grain, the area where rancidity occurs. Unfortunately, this is also where most of the nutrient value lies. The most valuable part of the grain is removed because of its vulnerability to rancidity, and we are left to consume the least nutritious part – white flour. Thus the staple food of most people's diets – white bread – is devoid of most of its nutrient value, so much so that, by law, some vitamins and minerals have to be put back into the bread. According to the bread manufacturers, this makes it as good as the original product. However, the replacements are inadequate and not in their natural form or balance, and the natural fibre content is not present.

Table 6: Comparison of 1972 and 1979 studies of children's nutrient intake

Nutrient	Percentage of children getting less than RDA	
	1972	*1979*
Vitamin B1	7	26
Vitamin B2	—	11
Vitamin B6	16.5	47
Vitamin A	8	5
Vitamin C	8	8
Calcium	9	35

Such is the extent of this refining process that it has been discovered that, where white bread and other refined grains constitute a significant part of a person's diet, it is common for people to be mildly deficient in some essential nutrients. For example, a study was conducted in Michigan, U.S.A. on the dietary habits of primary-level school children in relation to the nutrients they were getting from the food they ate.[1] A comparison was made between children assessed in 1972 and 1979. It was found that, in 1979, a higher proportion of refined and processed foods was being eaten and this was reflected in the nutritional status of these children. In certain nutrients, there was a significantly higher number of children receiving less than the Recommended Daily Allowance (RDA) for those vitamins and minerals, as described in Table 6.

Inherent problems are also present in the chemical method of food preservation. Although manufacturers claim that these chemicals are perfectly safe, the simple fact remains that they are part of an ever-increasing chemical environment that our bodies are being forced to deal with.

Chemicals that are used as food preservatives are foreign substances that the human body was not evolved to cope with. Although laboratory studies may show them to be safe, no one can be sure of their long-term effects on humans. For instance, one drastic consequence of the consumption of these chemicals is becoming increasingly apparent. Some people have become highly allergic to the chemicals to which they are exposed, both internally and externally. Their bodies are not able to handle the increasing amounts of chemicals that reach them through food, air and water. (See next chapter.)

Marked nutritional losses occur when other methods of food

preservation are used. Freezing, canning, dehydration and irradiation all decrease the quality of the food. Quite simply, a price has to be paid if the food is not eaten in its fresh and natural state.

One unfortunate side effect of the development of the food chemical industry was the discovery that chemical or synthetic products could be made to mimic many of the tastes naturally found in food. Not only this, but they could be used to give food a seemingly natural flavour at a fraction of the cost involved in using the real food substance. Thus, the use of artificial flavours and colours in foods began in earnest. Foodstuffs could now be produced that tasted like the real thing, but without having to use the more expensive, less stable, natural components. And with the use of these chemicals, poorer quality food could be used by adding artificial flavours and colours to improve its taste and appearance, or the natural food could be used in smaller quantities by using chemical substitutes.

What a master stroke of technology! Here surely is science at its best, for it seems to have outsmarted and even superseded Nature herself. But, as we are now unfortunately discovering, there was one fatal mistake in this technological revolution. The naturally forming substances in foods, which produce their particular flavours and colours, are almost without exception completely harmless. Indeed, they are part of the integral structure of the food itself. But the chemical additives used to flavour and colour foods are in most cases unnatural, and in some instances, potentially hazardous. As with the chemical preservatives, there is the question of the long term effects of the consumption of these foreign substances.

Already, some of these chemicals have been removed because evidence has emerged to show that they are not as safe as was originally thought. For instance, a food colouring called Red 2, or *Amaranth*, was in wide use in the United States of America during the 1960s. But Russian studies done at the time indicated that Red 2 caused birth defects, foetal deaths and cancer in laboratory animals. Its use in the U.S.A. was subsequently curtailed, despite some strong resistance from the food colour manufacturers.[2] Unbelievably, Red 2 is still widely used in Australia to colour a great variety of foods.[3] Several other chemicals have been removed altogether or their use severely restricted as a result of studies showing them to be carcinogenic (cancer causing).

Each of these chemicals has been looked at in isolation and the effects of exposure assessed over a relatively short period of time, considering that humans may consume them for most of their lives. The long term, cumulative effects of all the chemicals that are consumed through food is unknown – if ever determined, the results may indeed be frightening. Some people are finding that their bodies cannot tolerate this chemical loading, and it is adversely affecting their behaviour, learning abilities and general disposition.

Good nutrition does not end with the avoidance of chemical additives. In fact, this is only the beginning, for the adulteration of previously good, wholesome foods has not only occurred through chemical means. Since the processing and refinement of grains severely depletes their nutritional value, whole (unrefined) grain products should be eaten in preference to those made with white flour. Great care also needs to be taken concerning the amount of sugar consumed.

Sugar cane, before it is refined, is an acceptable food, rich in many nutrients. But the extreme processing that it undergoes to produce white and 'raw' sugar makes it virtually devoid of any nutrients. It is an empty food, of value only for its sweetening ability. The consumption of sugar in most Western countries has reached astronomical proportions. In Australia for example, it was estimated that in 1982 around 53 kilograms of sugar was consumed for each person on a per capita basis. That is the alarming equivalent of one kilogram per week per person.

How could the consumption rate possibly be so high? Well, sugar has become a ubiquitous foodstuff, to the point that it is almost impossible to avoid it if commercially prepared foods are eaten. As well, it is used in much greater quantities than most people would suspect. For instance, a can of carbonated soft drink may contain up to half a cup of sugar, and some commercial fruit juices that use sugar for sweetening may have just as much. It is also used in foods that most people would not suspect as containing sugar – in many brands of wholemeal breads for example, and even in some cans of salad beans. When the different ways in which sugar is used are looked at, it is not at all surprising that so much is consumed.

What is so bad about sugar? The sugar industry would have you believe that it is a perfectly nutritious food that forms an essential part of our diet and they maintain that it is good for bodily energy production. However, since it has been refined to the point where it contains so few nutrients, sugar could be said to be of no nutritional value. The only thing in its favour, apart from its obvious sweetening capacity, is that it does help in providing the body with energy but even this is only partially true.

In fact, sugar is not a good form of 'energy food'. The brain has a need for glucose far out of proportion to its size. Although it is a relatively small organ, it requires around 20 per cent of the available glucose that circulates in the blood. This glucose is the end product of the breakdown of starches. The blood glucose (or sugar) level needs to be constantly maintained at an optimum level, so that the brain can receive what it needs. When white or raw sugar is consumed, it is absorbed very quickly, because of its highly refined state. As a result, it rapidly sends the blood sugar level higher, giving a burst of energy – the thing that sugar is meant to be good for. But it is used up just as quickly as it is absorbed, and the blood sugar level rapidly drops as a result. Thus the energy boost is not maintained.

Even though this burst of energy is short lived, wouldn't it be possible to keep it at a high level simply by eating more sugar? Unfortunately, it is not as easy as this, for there is a potential danger in consuming too much sugar. The blood sugar level should be fairly constant, and if it is continually going up and down as sugar is taken in, burnt up and then replaced, problems can develop. One danger is that the blood sugar level may drop very quickly following a sudden and rapid rise, and it then could fall lower than the minimum level the brain needs for normal operation. Since at this point the brain is not receiving enough glucose, the body's functions may be adversely affected, and it may result in symptoms such as fatigue, anxiety, depression, headaches, insomnia, and a general decrease in performance.

Instead of following a roller coaster course, the blood sugar level needs to be kept at a constant level. This can be achieved by eating foods that contain complex rather than simple carbohydrates. Foods such as wholemeal bread and other whole grains, nuts, and other high protein foods such as legumes, dairy products, eggs, fish and meat should be eaten. These foods are *slowly* broken down, and supply a more constant source of glucose than refined, sweet foods, thereby avoiding a sudden rise and fall of the blood sugar level.

Salt is another food that is over-consumed by many people. It is found to be prevalent in processed foods, often in extremely large amounts. Thus, it is very easy to consume more salt than is good for the body, even without adding it to food while eating. It is now thought that excessive salt intake is one of the major factors contributing to high blood pressure and heart disease. Most natural foods contain enough sodium to supply the body's needs – extra salt does not need to be added.

There are many other warnings that we could give about foods that you may have been happily eating until now. However, as this is not a nutrition book. It is better that you also read books solely devoted to the subject of nutrition. There is a reading list at the end of this chapter to encourage and assist you. We recommend that you study some of these books.

So where does this leave you now? You may want to change your family's diet, but may not know how to go about it. Earlier, we said that foods which taste good aren't necessarily good for you. However, this doesn't mean that nutritious foods don't taste very nice. On the contrary, there are enough delicious natural foods to keep most gourmets content for life.

This is the challenge of good nutrition – to discover some of the many nutritious foods that are appealing to the palate, and to learn exciting ways of preparing them. It's a challenging new world that will require some different ideas concerning preparation and meal structures, but the effort will be well worthwhile – not only for better health, but also for improved taste.

Children usually adapt better to a change of diet than do adults. However, you need to be careful in the way you go about it. When your new diet is introduced, certain rules about which foods can and can't be eaten need to be established and strictly adhered to. If the children are old enough, the reasons for the changes in their diet should be carefully explained, and they should be given lots of positive reinforcement for eating the right foods. Be prepared for complaints in the first couple of weeks as it is human nature to react adversely to change. But as the pleasures of the new foods are discovered, the grumbles should give way to appreciation.

Again, since this is not a nutrition book, space does not permit us to discuss the many things you can do with the new diet, but the recommended books should give you many good ideas. Some of the foods that should be part of a good nutrition program include whole grains such as wheat, oats, barley, rye and brown rice; high protein legumes such as soy beans and chick peas; fresh nuts; a wide variety of fresh fruits and vegetables; and dairy foods and animal products, although both these should be used in moderation.

The use of vitamin and mineral supplements is another aspect of nutrition that needs to be considered when dealing with brain injured children. The potential benefit of their use was demonstrated in a 1981 study conducted by Ruth Harrell[4], a doctor in the U.S.A. Harrell added eleven vitamins and eight minerals to the otherwise unchanged diets of sixteen mentally retarded children. To eliminate other possible influences, no alteration was made to the children's schooling, socialization or lifestyle. Also in this study, some of the children were given 'placebo tablets', capsules containing no supplements – no child was aware if he was receiving the real tablet or the placebo.

The results of this study were quite significant: during the first four months, the group receiving the placebo tablets made an average gain of 1.1 on their IQ score, while the group receiving the supplements gained an average 10.8 points. Over an eight-month period, the average increase in the IQ score of the supplement children was around 16 points.

In fact, four children increased their IQ scores by 30 to 40 points, and they were able to be transferred from special to normal classes in their schools. One fifteen-year-old achieved normal grade level performance, but when taken off the supplements, her IQ regressed to less than 50. As well, an increase in weight gain and more rapid increase in height was noted in some of the children taking the supplements.

The number of children involved in this study is too small to make its results statistically valid. However, the findings cannot be ignored, for they point very clearly to the importance of vitamin and mineral supplements for brain injured children. Such treatment should be directed by a nutritionally orientated doctor or health practitioner, as the type and amounts of supplements to be used are specific to each individual child.

Special note on breastfeeding and brain injured babies

Breastfeeding your brain injured baby is one of the best things you can do for him. It provides optimum nutrition, immunity to disease and infection, and emotional nurturing. In breast milk, Nature has provided the most perfect food available for the newborn. Except in rare cases, there is no substitute that can better this food.

Recently, there has been an explosion of medical and scientific research highlighting the importance of breastfeeding. You can keep up-to-date on the latest findings by joining the Nursing Mothers Association of Australia (NMAA), or the international La Leche League. These organizations offer practical support and instruction in all aspects of breastfeeding, including the breast-feeding of babies with disabilities. They also provide access to reading material on breastfeeding, offer counselling on specific problems, and have a well developed social network of nursing mothers.

Breastfeeding a brain injured baby may be more difficult than in normal circumstances. The baby may suck less efficiently, have poor muscle tone, be more prone to respiratory infections, or may even have to be woken for feeds or during feeding. Despite all of the problems that may arise, it is best to persist for as long as possible. In some cases, the baby may eventually become a good feeder, but simply needs more time to develop this skill. With an understanding of the importance of breastfeeding, the reasons why a mother should keep trying to establish a good feeding pattern become quite clear.

For instance, Dr Peter Hartmann, a senior lecturer in biochemistry at the University of Western Australia and an NMAA adviser, says: 'We have looked at the records of 10,000 deliveries in our maternity hospital; in thirteen parameters, the babies that are breastfed are significantly better off than those who are bottle fed, and there is no parameter in which the babies who are bottlefed are better off than breastfed babies.'[5]

According to Dr K. R. Kamath[6], head of the Department of Gastroenterology, Royal Alexandra Hospital for Children, Sydney, the nutritional advantages of breast milk are best understood by comparing it to its nearest rival which is sometimes used for feeding babies – cow's milk. Cow's milk has at least two-and-one-half to three times as much protein as human milk. It has three times as much salt, four times as much calcium and six times as much phosphorus. Dr Kamath points out that the higher levels of these nutrients in cow's milk may be deleterious to the human baby. Apart from its nutrient superiority, Dr Kamath discusses the anti-infective role and possible anti-allergic effect of human milk. The special protein called immunoglobulin A which helps the body fight infection is present in only very low concentration, if at all, in the first weeks of life. The baby receives immunoglobulin A, along with other essential antibodies, through his mother's breast milk, and thus a means for fighting infections that the baby may be exposed to is established. As well, a baby fed breast milk exclusively is not exposed to any foods that his immature immune system may be unable to cope with; therefore he his less likely to develop allergies to foods in general.

Apart from the health and nutritional advantages of breastfeeding, the following considerations are also very important:

● Bonding with your brain injured child is important for his welfare and for your acceptance of him as part of the family. Breastfeeding helps stimulate that bonding, and provides emotional warmth and physical closeness for mother and child. It is a special relationship.

● It provides optimum stimulation of the mouth, lips and tongue which can help with low muscle tone babies, and it provides an important early foundation for speech development.

● It guards against obesity. A brain injured child with motor problems who has excess weight may have more difficulty learning to move.

The symmetrical stimulation that takes place during breastfeeding helps to develop both sides of the brain. The baby is held on alternate sides for feeding, something that rarely happens with bottle feeding. When the baby is on the mother's left breast, the left eye, being away from her body, works harder than the right side. When the baby is on the right breast, the opposite applies.

Special mention needs to be made of situations where a baby may be separated from his mother after birth. When this occurs, it is best that the baby receives expressed milk that has come from his mother rather than from a pooled source, if this is possible. Research has shown the levels of various nutrients in breast milk varies quite considerably, depending on the age of the baby being breastfed[7]. Thus, it would be inappropriate for a three-day-old baby to receive expressed milk that contains milk from a mother who was breastfeeding a six-month-old. This is especially important in the case of premature babies, as the difference between the composition of pre-term and pooled milk is even greater than the difference between full-term and pooled milk[8].

Three currently available books that are particularly helpful for breastfeeding brain injured children are: *You Can Breastfeed Your Baby . . . Even in Special Situations* by Dorothy Patricia Brewster (Rodale Press, Emmaus, U.S.A.), and *How to be a Parent of a Handicapped Child and Survive* by Kerry Kenihan (Penguin, Ringwood, Australia), *Breast Feeding Matters* by Maureen Mirchin (Alma Publications).

Recommended Reading List of Books Advising on Nutrition

Airola, Paavo, *Airola Diet and Cookbook*, Health Plus Publishers, Phoenix, U.S.A., 1981

Airola, Paavo, *Are You Confused?* Health Plus Publishers, Phoenix, U.S.A., 1971

Airola, Paavo, *Everywoman's Book*, Health Plus Publishers, Phoenix, U.S.A., 1979

Buchman, Ellen, *Recipes for a Small Planet*, Ballantine, New York, U.S.A., 1973

Katzen, Mollie, *Moosewood Cookbook*, Ten Speed Press, Berkeley, U.S.A., 1977

Katzen, Mollie, *The Enchanted Broccoli Forest*, Ten Speed Press, Berkeley, U.S.A., 1982

Smith, Lendon, *Feed Your Kids Right*, Delta, New York, U.S.A., 1979

CHAPTER TWENTY-SIX

Allergies

A Missing Link in Brain Injury – the Unsuspected Brain Allergy Connection
By Dr Marshall Mandell *

My investigation of the profound effects of commonly encountered brain and bodywide allergies in a group of brain injured volunteers, and over 4000 patients with a wide variety of physical and mental disorders, has shown that an accurate diagnosis and proper management of their hidden allergies has given many of them a greatly enhanced quality of life, both physically and mentally. My research concerning the demonstrable and reproducible allergic reactions of brain injured patients led to a startling discovery – that many brain injured children and adults have a very important, but heretofore unrecognized, allergic or allergy-like state of vulnerability in, or adjacent to, the site(s) of the original injury in their nervous systems.

These vulnerable areas, which I have named 'biologic weak spots', are frequently or continuously undergoing previously unsuspected allergic reactions to commonly encountered dietary and environmental substances that have significant effects on these areas of the brain. Along with their cerebral reactions, many brain injured individuals also have other kinds of unrecognized internal allergic reactions that occur in other areas of their bodies. The overall effect of these hidden and uncontrolled allergies is to cause intermittent or unending symptoms that make the problems related to the brain injury, and any other existing disorders, much

---

* Dr Marshall Mandell, M.D., D.A.B.P, D.A.B.A.I., F.A.C.A., F.S.C.E., F.I.A.M., F.I.A.P.M. is a leading U.S.A. allergist and author of *Dr Mandell's 5-Day Allergy Relief System, Dr Mandell's Lifetime Arthritis Relief System, The Mandell's 'It's Not Your Fault You're Fat' Diet* and numerous scientific papers.

worse – often very much worse than the original brain injury is capable of making them.

As you will see as this chapter progresses, the reactions caused by exposures to substances that the patient is allergic to are indistinguishable from many of the symptoms which in the past have always been directly related to brain injury. For instance, many parents of brain injured children have observed that there are often marked fluctuations in their child's day-to-day neuromuscular activities, mental ability and emotional state. One day the child is good, next day he is not so good, sometimes being unable to do the things he could do the day before. Usually this dilemma has been attributed to the child's condition – as being simply part of the problem – for one of the common characteristics of brain injured children has always been this previously misinterpreted variation in performance. But, as the exciting results of my research have shown, problems such as this may in fact be aggravated or even caused by the patient's allergic reactions.

This discovery has opened the door to a much brighter future for many brain injured individuals. We can diagnose and prevent or minimize the effects of these heretofore unsuspected allergic reactions, reactions that may adversely affect the physical abilities of a brain injured person, decrease the intellectual abilities of a so-called mentally retarded person, worsen the seizure pattern of an epileptic, or make it even more difficult for a slow learner to keep up with his classmates.

The symptoms due to 'brain allergies' may be constant, almost continuous, or they may come and go. This is because the allergic reactions that underlie the symptoms are caused by different kinds of exposures to the reaction-causing substances. Constant or chronic symptoms result from continuous or closely spaced exposures to the offending substances, and intermittently appearing symptoms are due to intermittent contact with the culprits.

If the symptoms come and go, we can be certain that we are dealing with a reversible disease process, or the symptoms would never clear up. This is very good news to those who have wondered why there were good and bad days that no one seemed to understand. You must always keep in mind the fact that reversible brain malfunctions are evidence of an underlying process that can often be identified and controlled.

These brain allergies may occur in otherwise normal people who suffer from the well-known allergic disorders like hives, eczema, seasonal hay fever and bronchial asthma. But, these common allergies may or may not be present in cases of nervous system allergy. If these common skin and respiratory tract allergies were present in every individual who had nervous system allergies, this close association would have been observed and the brain injury-allergy connection would have been suspected, searched for, and probably found many years ago. The connection was overlooked and remained an unrecognized entity because these conditions very often occur independently of each other.

A very broad spectrum of allergic, toxic, and allergy-like sensitivity reactions often occur in the central nervous systems of millions of vulnerable individuals whose biological or biochemical makeup somehow predisposes them to having such reactions. These reactions take place with great frequency because the human brain is continuously exposed to an unavoidable and unending environmental reservoir of biologically active substances from many sources.

As you will see from the accompanying illustration, many of the major causes of these commonly encountered nervous system malfunctions are unavoidable because these substances – food, water and air – are essential to our survival. As long as we live, there will

1 The unsmiling man locked in the triangle of bio-ecologic illness
Many forms of physical and mental disorders are caused by unavoidable substances in our environment that are essential to our survival

```
                            { }
WATER      —  \/[ | ]\/  —   AIR
                  [ _ ]
                 /     \
               _ |      | _
```

_____

FOOD & BEVERAGES

be no end to our possible illness-evoking exposures to whatever health-affecting substances our inescapable contacts with food, water and air may bring into our bodies from the outside world.

On numerous occasions, each one of us is exposed to airborne allergenic particles such as house dust, animal danders, seasonal pollens, indoor and outdoor moulds and microscopic parts that come from the bodies of many species of insects. There is additional contact with hundreds or thousands of chemical agents in the form of powders or fumes that will pollute the atmosphere within our homes, at the places of our employment, in the school environment, during the course of recreational activities, and in many public places in which numerous possible causes of environmental (eco-logic) disorders are encountered.

Inhaled particles like pollens and moulds will adhere to the moist surfaces of the nose and throat and some of the allergically active materials they contain will go into solution (dissolve) in this moisture and be absorbed into the system. Other particles that are trapped in the mucus on these surfaces will be swallowed and processed by the digestive tract as if they had been eaten. When they are absorbed from the intestines, they will enter the circulation and be transported throughout the body, exposing all of the potential allergy reaction sites in every system. Vapours and fumes, including combustion products, enter the lungs and pass through the walls of the air sacs into the blood and also reach all of the body's potential reaction sites as shown in the illustration on page 000.

It is important to realize that the brain has the richest blood supply of any organ in the body. Consequently, it is heavily exposed to all of the active and potential allergic, toxic and metabolic offenders that are present in the vulnerable individual's diet and environment.

The normal functions of the brain cells of children and adults who cannot tolerate these substances for any reason, will be interfered with, and these adverse cerebral (brain) reactions may trigger, aggravate, or perpetuate familiar nervous system signs or symptoms that characterize each person's specific disability. These brain reactions may cause very severe responses because the brain is an extremely complex, delicately balanced structure – one of the great marvels of creation or evolution – that controls many interrelated functions with miraculous precision. Because of its exquisite degree of sensitivity, the brain is easily disturbed by the

2 *Allergic reactions causing multiple physical and mental symptoms*
Bodywide distribution of environmental substances

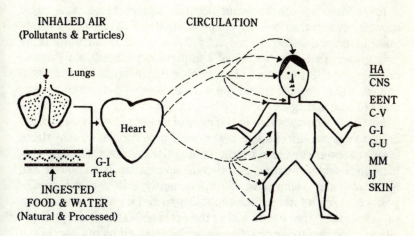

INHALED AIR
(Pollutants & Particles)

CIRCULATION

Lungs

Heart

G-I
Tract

INGESTED
FOOD & WATER
(Natural & Processed)

HA
CNS

EENT
C-V

G-I
G-U

MM
JJ
SKIN

HA   = Headache
CNS   = Central Nervous System
EENT = Eyes, Ears, Nose & Throat
C-V   = Cardiovascular System
G-I   = Gastrointestinal Tract
G-U   = Genitourinary Tract
MM   = Muscles
JJ   = Joints

effects of outside influences and extremely important physical, mental, emotional and behavioural changes will occur following an exposure to dietary and/or environmental offenders.

I have repeatedly observed significant variations in the chronic and intermittent physical and mental-emotional manifestations of several thousand patients who have many forms of nervous system disorders. The volunteer group of brain injured children and young adults were among these individuals. The articulate brain injured and non-brain injured patients, and their parents or spouses, have frequently made this same observation. They reported their frustration with their unpredictable and puzzling ailments. They stated that, at times, their neurologic disorders had been a slightly to moderately uncomfortable and relatively minor handicap that was 'inconvenient'. At other times, they had experienced painful and incapacitating flare-ups of their conditions that seemed to 'come from out of nowhere'.

In addition to the abovementioned unpredictable, seemingly spontaneous, variations in their ailments, I have deliberately brought on numerous episodes of the very same symptoms by giving each patient a series of symptom-duplicating, sublingual, provocative allergy tests.* I interpreted this information as clinical evidence that demonstrated the existence of an extremely important biologic (allergic or allergy-like, and/or metabolic-biochemical-nutritional) predisposition of the cells of an injured or dysorganized brain to sustain undesirable reactions. I also concluded that these brain reactions caused cerebral malfunctions characterized by various undesirable mental, emotional, perceptual, behavioural and neuromuscular symptoms. This frequently encountered predisposition to react (state of susceptibility to dietary and environmental substances) that exists within the brain cells that undergo these allergic and metabolic reactions is well explained by my concept of 'biologic weak spots'.

These weak spots are reaction-prone cells and their associated pathways that are vulnerable (allergically and metabolically susceptible) because they are either irritable, incompletely recovered (with impaired functioning from residual damage), or neuro-developmentally dysorganized. I believe that the weak spots which are associated with brain injury are created in the following manner: with the passing of time, the structures at the site of the brain injury will have 'recovered' as completely as they possibly can. The most severely damaged 'central' area of the injury will have undergone permanent, irreversible destruction that is surrounded by a peripheral zone that consists of irritable and partially or almost com-

---

* A sublingual (under-the-tongue) test is performed by placing carefully measured doses of allergy-testing solutions on the floor of the mouth, directly behind the lower front teeth. There is a large group of thin-walled capillary blood vessels (the sublingual plexus) very close to the surface in this area. Drugs like nitroglycerine (given for heart disease), chemical solutions, and various kinds of allergy test extracts are very rapidly absorbed into the circulation from this site. They are carried in the blood to all of the allergically or otherwise vulnerable areas in the body, usually causing symptoms within one or two minutes.

pletely healed brain tissue. The overall functioning of the cells in the peripheral zone is impaired and these abnormal, less resistant cells become the sites in which adverse reactions are initiated much more readily.

In cases of hay fever, an allergic person's biologic weak spots are the pollen-sensitive tissues of the upper respiratory tract and the conjunctival membrane (surface of the eye and lining of the lids) which react to spring and summer pollens. Contact with an offending tree, grass or weed pollen will cause the typical allergic symptoms of sneezing with an itchy, runny or blocked nose; ear, and throat symptoms, along with runny, itchy, red eyes. The brain injured person's vulnerable weak spots are located in and adjacent to the site of the injury. Cerebral weak spots consist of irritable or partially recovered brain cells that function in an almost normal manner.

My laboratory technicians and I have evoked thousands of familiar cerebral and neuromuscular reactions during the numerous symptom-duplicating sublingual tests that we have performed with food extracts. The results of this testing were subsequently confirmed with single-food ingestion challenges that induced the same symptoms. In my opinion, these observations have firmly established food allergy as a significant factor in central nervous system disorders. The greatly improved level of functioning and the much improved comfort that resulted from the elimination of food offenders identified by provocative laboratory and ingestion testing are undeniable clinical proof that brain allergies make the symptoms of brain injury much worse than they would be if these reactions did not occur. The illustration on page **000** illustrates my concept of biologic weak spots.

In addition to this concept of residual areas of vulnerable brain tissues at the sites of cerebral injuries, I have also concluded that cerebral 'short circuits' caused by neurophysiologic stresses play an important role in the genesis of cerebral allergies.

I believe that biologically unstable allergy reaction sites are created in the brain if a child fails to pass through the entire sequence of normal development which is achieved by progressing through increasingly complex stages of neurologic maturation. The failure of a child to adequately experience these learning and stabilizing influences leads to a state of physiologic immaturity in certain structures of the nervous system which become functional

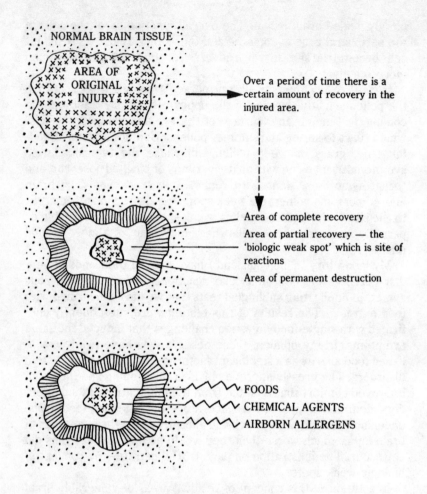

NORMAL BRAIN TISSUE

AREA OF ORIGINAL INJURY

Over a period of time there is a certain amount of recovery in the injured area.

Area of complete recovery

Area of partial recovery — the 'biologic weak spot' which is site of reactions

Area of permanent destruction

FOODS

CHEMICAL AGENTS

AIRBORN ALLERGENS

The biologic weak spot at the brain injury site

weak spots. I visualize these weak spots as anatomically normal areas of the brain that malfunction because they have not been adequately stimulated in the manner that is required to establish their normal function.

Normal neurologic organization is the final result of having the nerve control centres – and their associated pathways – perform the same functions repeatedly until the closely integrated patterns of nerve impulses have become sets of automatically learned responses, responses that are performed smoothly and rapidly whenever they are called upon. Neurologic dysorganization is the often disabling condition that exists when the nervous system has not followed its normal developmental progression. I believe that the immature or dysorganized brain areas malfunction when called upon to perform their often complex activities. Reactions occur in these areas because because they are 'out of alignment' and are easily disturbed by inciting agents that do not affect a stable, normally organized brain.

The Discovery of the Brain Injury-Allergy Connection

My realization that a link existed between brain injury and allergy began quietly one afternoon in my office when I was seeing yet another patient seeking relief from respiratory allergies. The experiences of that day captured my imagination, and started me on a fascinating and absorbing study that eventually demonstrated how the condition of brain injury is often made much worse by the effects of brain allergies.

John, a twenty-six-year-old from Florida, was different from all the other allergy patients I had seen up until that time, a difference that was immediately obvious as he limped into my office. He had the familiar history of 'treatment-resistant' nasal, sinus and bronchial allergies, but in addition to these problems he also had suffered brain injury at birth which had left him with the symptoms of mild cerebral palsy. His whole left side was involved, hence the limp when he walked and the way his left hand hung limply from his forearm which was held in an awkward, elevated position in front of his body. In addition, his facial muscles and his speech were affected.

As expected, my allergy laboratory technicians were able to reproduce all of his familiar respiratory tract symptoms by giving him a series of single-blind sublingual provocative tests with solutions made from foods, inhalants and chemical agents.* These test-

* When tests are performed by the single-blind technique, the person being tested is not told which substances are being given to him. This procedure is followed to avoid the possibility that he may be consciously or unconsciously influenced by such information, which might possibly affect the test results.

evoked allergic reactions in his upper and lower respiratory tract identified the causes of his nasal, sinus and bronchial allergies.

In addition to aggravating his usual respiratory symptoms, the allergy tests caused reactions that initially surprised me greatly – they actually made his cerebral palsy symptoms worse. Now, with the benefit of hindsight, I realize that I should not have been so startled by what happened to John, but at the time it seemed an amazing discovery. The unexpected neurologic symptoms induced by the testing included the following: extreme fatigue to the point of falling asleep, intense headache, severe dizziness, visual blurring that made reading very difficult, a sense of intoxication and unreality, nervousness, an inner shaky feeling, uncomfortable generalized tingling, and moderate aching tenseness of the back muscles. A severe spasm of the flexor muscles controlling the fingers of his left hand made it impossible for him to open his hand for ten minutes.

These were symptoms that John had lived with all his life, and had accepted as the usual and expected discomforts that accompany cerebral palsy. John and his parents had been told that 'this is the way things are for cerebral palsied people', and no one paid any serious attention to what was believed to be an inevitable consequence of having this condition. But John's test results showed that this was not the case. The subsequent treatment of John's allergies improved many of his cerebral palsy symptoms, for as well as feeling better, the functions of the affected parts of his body were definitely improved.

I became very excited with the thought that a significant portion of brain injury-related problems may have a connection to allergy rather than just to the brain injury itself. The revelations that unfolded that day also fitted in nicely with my concept of biologic weak spots, because John's cerebral palsy manifestations got worse with provocative testing. This strongly suggested that the allergy reaction sites in his brain must be intimately related to the original injury sites, otherwise John's cerebral palsy symptoms would not have been caused or exacerbated by testing.

Suddenly, a whole new area of allergy treatment became apparent, and in an attempt to confirm my initial findings, I established a research project to investigate the apparent relationship between brain injury and allergy. Twenty-five people were involved in this study, and in all of these cases the primary manifestation of their brain injury was cerebral palsy. Each person was given a comprehensive series of allergic challenges, and in each case these tests caused reactions that produced familiar symptoms of their cerebral palsy. This research project yielded a set of remarkable findings that went far beyond my greatest expectations. Can you imagine my excitement when I realized that each person had test-evoked cerebral reactions that were identical to their lifelong cerebral palsy symptoms? I was convinced that these test results indicated it was highly likely that many of the painful and disabling effects of brain injury could be alleviated or even eradicated by relatively simple drug-free and surgery-free ecologic management.

One of the most exciting aspects of this investigation was that each of the brain injured people we studied had physical and/or mental reactions to foods and environmental substances. Instead of reacting to just one or two foods, chemicals or environmental substances, most of them reacted to many, and in some cases most, of the tests. This showed that the allergic reactions in this group of brain injured people were not random or isolated, but in fact formed an extremely complex allergy picture. Some of their most important reactions to testing were:

A nine year old girl became very aggressive as she reacted to pineapple extract. Automobile exhaust, house dust, aspergillis (mould), and honey made her lethargic. Tomato disturbed her coordination. Apricot made her dizzy. Egg and cheddar cheese made her legs jerk.

An eight year old girl had one of her usual 'blackouts' from her test with the mould, penicillium. Egg, peanut, brewer's yeast, and petroleum alcohol (chemical ethanol) made her sleepy. Ethanol also provoked a typical episode of frustrated crying with biting and scratching.

A three year old girl had a mild seizure from house dust mites which also caused her to fall asleep. She also had seizures from ethanol and tree pollen extract. Pea extract tightened the muscles in her arms, and she became disoriented from a test with a garden spray. There was nasal congestion from chlorine, wheat, and a mixture of weed pollens.

A twelve year old girl became sleepy from beef, had a familiar kind of 'startle' spasm from pork, and developed nasal congestion from egg, grape, baker's yeast and navy beans.

Other patients reacted to their provocative tests with symptoms that occurred in other parts of the body as well as in the nervous system. Their symptoms are listed below:

Silliness	Depression
Slurred speech	Disorientation
Extreme irritability	Euphoria
Loss of coordination	Hysterical behaviour
Muscle spasms	Neck stiffness
Anger	Unable to hold head up
Agitated behaviour	Arms flapping
Loud vocalizing	Uncontrollable leg shaking with
Fighting	difficulty in standing
Screaming	and walking
Kicking	Sore throat
Hyperactivity	Rectal pain
Staring spells	Vaginal pain
Loss of balance	Drooling

As expected, no particular food, inhalant, or chemical caused the same symptoms in each patient. Each substance provoked different reactions in different patients, just as they did with all of my other patients who have various kinds of allergic disorders. The manifestations of sensitivity to dietary and environmental incitants are unique, patient-specific reactions. This investigation showed that a wide variety of substances to which all of us are frequently exposed, can affect the functioning and general health of people who have cerebral palsy. As well as showing that allergies frequently aggravated the symptoms of brain injury, by means of this research project I was able to demonstrate that by treating the allergies, there were corresponding improvements in many of the problems thought to be solely caused by brain injury. Conservative, non-invasive, biologically sound 'anti-allergy' measures were directed toward the test-identified dietary/environmental factors that made the problems of brain injury much worse than they had to be. Some improvements reported by patients included:

Reduced muscle pain	More relaxed
Increased limb mobility	Improved sleep
Decreased spasticity	Positive personality changes
Improved balance	Decreased fatigue
Decreased seizures	Decreased irritability
Decreased hyperactivity	A happier state of mind

At the other end of the spectrum of brain injury are the children with reading and learning problems who may also be hyperactive and mood swingers. Just as with cerebral palsy, I have found that allergies can severely affect the performance of these children. To demonstrate how they can be affected, I have used handwriting as a reliable reference point, since the ability to write represents an extremely complex neurologic activity that, because of its complexity, is more vulnerable to any slight disturbance in the brain. The following examples clearly demonstrate this point:

Laura

This seven year old's life was characterized by great variations in her physical activity and mental ability. She was very bright, with an IQ of 120, but at times she lapsed into a state where she would lose her memory, be unable to hold a normal conversation, and wander aimlessly around her school, unsure of where she actually was. Despite her intelligence, her penmanship, spelling and sentence structure were very poor most of the time. However, at other times she was like a completely different child, resembling what her parents liked to call 'the real Laura'. When I tested Laura for allergies, I found that she had very strong reactions to cow's milk and two common household moulds, fusarium and aspergillis. Apart from causing many other symptoms, these reactions had a drastic affect on her handwriting, as can be seen below:

Usual writing	Laura Belanger
Reaction to milk	Jauradehger
Reaction to Fusarium	pejag gr
Reaction to Aspergillus	Lautanger

Cheryl

This highly allergic ten-year-old girl suffered from hay fever, hives, asthma, and severe reactions to bee and wasp stings. She often became very confused or completely disorientated after being exposed to the fumes and combustion products of various petroleum distillates, as can be seen in her reaction to petroleum-derived ethyl alcohol.

Normal drawing and letter writing

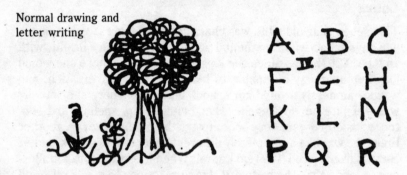

Drawing and letter writing while reacting to the petroleum-derived ethyl alcohol test for allergy-like sensitivity to chemicals.

Andy (nine years old)

Andy was best described as a lovable, irritable, hyperactive, learning-disabled 'wild man'. He had been pushed through school and had major speech, reading and writing problems. His behaviour was wildly erratic, and at times he was uncontrollable. He had severe eczema, and his skin was badly scarred. On testing, he was found to react to many foods, chemicals and environmental agents, and some of his reactions included increased hyperactivity, headache, withdrawn and moody behaviour, nausea, abdominal pain, hysteria, and many tantrums. He was asked to write his name and the numbers from one to ten during each of his sublingual tests. Some of the changes that occurred in his handwriting are shown on page **000**.

Normal handwriting   *Andrew Alexander*   *1 2 3 4 5 6 7 8 9 10*

Reaction to orange   *andy alexander*

Rice   *andy alexander 1 2 3 4 5 6 7 8 9 10*

Celery   *andy alexander 1 2 3 4 5 6*

Onion   *alexander andy 1 2 3 4 5 6*

Dust   *andrew alexander*

Chlorine   *andy alexander*

Food Preservatives   *andy andy*

Red food colour   *andy andy*   *alexander andy*

Automobile exhaust   *1 2 3 4 5 6 7 8 9 10*   *alexander*

Jason

An eleven-year-old boy with symptoms of frequent fatigue and restless behaviour

Usual handwriting

Jason Tunick   12345678910

Reactions to three challenges with soybean extract

Reactions to three challenges with egg extract

Jenny

A nine-year-old girl unable to do her schoolwork well despite above average intelligence

Usual handwriting

Jenny Field   12345678910

Reaction to roquefort cheese extract

Reaction to curvullaria (mould)

Reaction to cigarette smoke

Some General Comments About Allergies

In any discussion on allergies, it is necessary to look at the important allergic differences that exist between the closely related members of the plant and animal kingdoms that either constitute our food supply, or float about in the air as pollens, moulds or animal danders.

Certain foods belong to particular food families, with each food in a particular family sharing a botanical relationship with all the other foods of that family. For instance, oranges, grapefruit, lemons and limes are all members of the citrus family, but these foods are not identical. In most food families each food has a unique identity that makes it allergically distinct from everything else even though it may share some common factor(s) with the other closely related species of fruit or vegetables in its botanic family, or the meats, poultry or seafoods in its zoologic family. On the other hand, there are some very closely related cereal grains such as wheat, rye and barley, and mustard family vegetables like cabbage, brussels sprouts, cauliflower and broccoli that are now considered to be 'allergically identical'.

Sweeping generalizations cannot be made about avoiding certain foods that are related to each other. Just because a person is allergic to oranges does not automatically mean that he will react to the other members of the same food family as oranges. Even if he is allergic to several related foods, his reactions to each food might involve different bodily parts or systems and cause different symptoms.

Sometimes advice is given such as 'avoid nuts, spices and seafood'. But there is no specific nut family – peanuts, a *legume,* are not related in any way to an almond, a member of the *plum* family, or a pecan, part of the *walnut* family. There are all kinds of 'spices' in many different plant families. 'Seafood' includes an enormous number of allergically distinctive species of marine life, with the only common thread connecting them all being that they just happen to live in the same ocean, the same way that monkeys, elephants, snakes and grasshoppers live on dry land.

The same applies for environmental substances. A person with hay fever or internal pollen allergies may be very allergic to short ragweed pollen, but he may not react to pollen from the tall ragweed plant. The pollen of white oak trees may make him miserable, but the black oak or pin oak may not bother him at all. Kentucky blue grass may cause headache and fatigue, Canada blue grass might make him sneeze and cough, and annual blue grass could cause intense itching of the throat and palate and also block his ears and sinuses.

Every substance is unique, and every allergic person is unique. There is no room for guesswork in the diagnosis or management of an allergy. The specific role of each food or offending environmental substance has to be determined. One must not assume that all members of a particular biologic family or group of related chemicals will cause the same reactions – or any reaction – in a particular individual.

Another factor that needs to be carefully considered when food allergies are investigated is the frequency of exposure to each food. Some of the most common foods that people react to include dairy products, wheat and eggs. This does not mean that these are 'bad' foods for allergic people. They are major culprits because they are among the most commonly eaten foods in many people's diets. Meals containing an allergic individual's dietary offenders create a 'reservoir' or 'stockpile' of allergens in the digestive tract. These symptom-causing food culprits are continuously absorbed into the circulation during the digestive process, and they often cause prolonged symptoms since they remain in the bloodstream for a long time after they have been absorbed through the intestinal walls. The allergic reaction sites in the very sensitive braincells of brain injured and neurologically dysorganized people are exposed to food allergens for many hours or several days until the products of digestion have been utilized or excreted. If these offending foods are then consumed too frequently, symptoms may be chronic because the body may be almost continuously exposed to the reaction-evoking substances.

There is an important 'dosage factor' that determines the duration and intensity of allergic cerebral and bodywide reactions. It is the biologic summation of the combined effects of the ingested food and beverage allergens along with the added effects of the chemical additives and contaminants present in the foods and beverages. The quantities consumed and the frequency of exposure to these reaction-inducing foods and food-associated chemical agents are very important.

A similar 'dosage factor' applies to the cerebral reactions that occur following a chemically susceptible person's exposure to the volatile, biologically-active chemical agents that pollute our indoor and outdoor atmosphere. The frequency, intensity and duration of these reactions depends on the level of atmospheric pollution and how often the airborne fumes or vapours enter the circulation through the lungs and immediately reach all parts of the body, including the brain.

One of the most important signs indicating the presence of cerebral allergies in a brain injured person is significant variation in that individual's neuromuscular performance, mental functioning and behaviour. Physical and mental-emotional signs and symptoms that come and go are strong evidence of the highly probable presence of a reversible and usually controllable 'allergy' or nutritional-metabolic disorder.

An unexpected or unpredictable period of good health or good performance, or a temporary worsening in any of these areas, is proof that an affected individual does not have irreversible or untreatable damage at the site(s) of the disorder. Common sense tells us that an area of permanent destruction cannot function as if it were normal tissue. A period of good performance guarantees that a function has not been lost, but is being interfered with. Such clinical evidence tells us that we must look very hard and not stop until we have found the cause(s) of the variable or intermittent manifestations.

Summary

I have had the fascinating and exciting privilege of discovering and investigating the extremely important connection between brain injury – or physiologic brain dysfunction – and those frequently associated cerebral/somatic allergies that very often aggravate the underlying condition by adding a heavy, but unnecessary, burden to the lives of the afflicted and those who love them and care for them.

My initial observations on the serious effects of brain and body-wide allergy in cerebral palsy in the case of John M., and the wonderful co-operation of my research volunteers and their parents, has made it possible for me to open the door to a very effective new allergy-oriented diagnostic and treatment approach to brain injuries and brain dysfunctions.

The successful outcome in the majority of the patients who I have seen in consultation, tested and treated to date are living proof that there is good reason for great hope for many. There are hundreds of thousands of handicapped individuals with completely or partially reversible physical and mental-emotional disorders who no longer need to patiently endure suffering that can be relieved by currently available medical skills. Some of my fellow clinical ecologists with whom I shared my findings have confirmed my original observations.

By first diagnosing and then controlling the previously unsuspected and undiagnosed brain and bodywide allergies of a group of brain injured people, I have found that it is possible to greatly improve their quality of life, as well as increase their functional ability. This has been accomplished by eliminating or decreasing the frequency and intensity of the preventable or treatable allergic reactions that cause, aggravate or perpetuate many of their physical and/or mental symptoms. This applies both to the reactions occurring in the brain, as well as the numerous disorders that allergies can cause in other body areas apart from the central nervous system.

When an allergic brain injured or neurologically dysorganized individual is fortunate enough to receive appropriate allergy treatment in conjunction with an intensive therapy programme based upon the principles described in this book, then he has a good chance of making significant progress. These two treatment modalities certainly complement each other.

CHAPTER TWENTY-SEVEN

Epilepsy

THROUGHOUT history, epilepsy has been a misunderstood and feared condition. In earlier times, it was thought to be associated with the power of the devil. Reference is made to this in the New Testament, where Matthew, Luke and Mark each describe epileptic children as being possessed by the devil or an evil spirit. The Hebrew word *nichpea* translates into English as: 'to be inverted, upset; to be overtaken by a demon, especially due to epilepsy'.

Today, Satan is no longer thought to be involved, but epilepsy is still considered to be an 'illness' of drastic consequences. Those who have witnessed a grand mal convulsion will testify to its frightening nature, and can understand why people once thought it to be the devil's work.

Although the current approach to this problem is somewhat more enlightened, epilepsy is still shrouded in mystery, and is probably one of the least understood of all medical conditions. As well, there is confusion regarding diagnosis, with many different labels being used to describe what is essentially the same problem. Terms such as seizures, fits, jerks, spasms, turns, and convulsions may be used in addition to epilepsy, the choice of label depending to a large degree on which part of the world the child lives in.

A major advance in the attempt to analyse the nature and cause of epilepsy occurred in 1929, with the invention of the electroencephalograph or EEG machine, a device capable of measuring the electrical rhythms of the brain. The EEGs of epileptics showed that different varieties of epileptic attacks are associated with abnormal electrical rhythms, each different in its character and location in the brain. This discovery led to the description of epilepsy as being a cerebral dysrhythmia, and it demonstrated that epilepsy was related to abnormal electrical activity in the brain.

This opinion still holds true today, and is in fact still the basis for the current understanding of this problem. According to Lord Brain[1], an eminent British neurologist: 'There seems no doubt, however, that whatever its immediate or remote cause, an epileptic attack is the manifestation of a paroxysmal discharge of abnormal electrical rhythms in some part of the brain.'

However, despite the importance of the discovery of abnormal electrical activity, there is still little concrete information as to the true nature of epilepsy. Referring again to Brain, he states: 'We do not yet understand the physiological relationship between the dysrhythmia and the epileptic attack, or the nature of the physio-chemical disturbance which causes the dysrhythmia.'

Dekaban[2], a neurologist in the United States of America, perhaps best describes the dilemma concerning epilepsy: 'In analysing the clinical manifestations, it must be remembered that epilepsy is a symptom-complex which is the expression of a variety of abnormal processes in the brain. Certain of these may be structural, some are metabolic, and still others are undetectable with present methods. The difficulty in analysing epileptic phenomena lies in the great complexity of the brain as an organ, and in the fact that an epileptic discharge may originate in any group of neurons. Since a great variety of brain structures subserve different functions, it is clear that at least the initial clinical manifestation of the seizure will vary, depending on the site of its origin. In this way, we deal with a multi-plicity of pathological lesions and a multiplicity of clinical expres-sions.'

One thing that is known about epilepsy is that it is not a disease. It is no more a disease in its own right than high blood pressure or fever. Rather, it is a symptom of whatever is the cause of the abnormal electrical activity in the brain. One of these causes can be brain injury. It is this *brain injury-related epilepsy* with which the present chapter is concerned, not epilepsy caused by other means.

Although the types of epilepsy resulting from brain injury vary greatly, ranging from severe grand mal attacks to very mild and infrequent petit mal episodes, the initial precipitating factor is in some way related to the brain injury. Just how brain injury results in epilepsy is not clearly understood, but it is thought that in some cases it may be caused by scar tissue left by the injury, or by a disturbance in the normal electrical activity in the brain caused by the injury itself.

A major step in the treatment of epilepsy was made with the

discovery that certain types of drugs (known collectively as anti-convulsants) sometimes diminished the severity and frequency of epileptic attacks. According to Brain (see note 1 above), there are two ways that these drugs control the epilepsy – by the inhibition of the discharge of abnormal neurons, and by the prevention of the spread of the discharge once it has occurred. It seems that the drugs stabilize the normal neuronal membrane, or they increase the level of GABA – a neurotransmitter (chemical messenger in the brain) that has an inhibiting effect on the abnormal neuronal discharge.

Even though the use of anti-convulsant medication can sometimes be effective in controlling epilepsy, it does not directly treat the cause of the problem. The medication acts in a symptomatic way by suppressing the abnormal neuronal activity – it does not treat the *cause* of these abnormal discharges. In some cases, even though the treatment is symptomatic, epilepsy can be completely eliminated by the use of medication.

According to Lord Brain, this occurs because the medication is able to secure an abolition of attacks for a sufficient period of time, thereby enabling the patient to lose what Brain refers to as the 'epileptic habit'. But in our experience, such complete success is uncommon with brain injured children, especially in the cases of children with severe brain injuries. Usually these children have to take medication on a long-term basis, with little thought being given to eventually being able to stop the drugs. In such cases, if the medication is not taken, the seizures usually return (if they had been eliminated by the medication), or they get worse (if they had only been partially controlled). This is a clear indication that the drugs were only suppressing the symptoms of the epilepsy.

Through experience, doctors have found that certain types of epilepsy respond better to particular anti-convulsant drugs, and in these cases it is relatively straightforward as to which medications should be prescribed. However, there are many cases where the epilepsy proves difficult to control. In these situations, a systematic trial and error approach is adopted – the drug thought most likely to succeed is tried first, then if this doesn't achieve the desired result, others are introduced as either substitutes or additions. With all of this, there are still some cases where the epilepsy remains only partially controlled, or can only be contained if high doses of medication are used.

Although essentially a symptomatic form of treatment, the use of anti-convulsant medication could be completely justified if there was no other way of treating epilepsy, and if the drugs used had little or no side effects. After all, no one wants to see a child having seizures. However, there *are* adverse effects from some of these drugs, and sometimes the effect can be quite debilitating. Most have a general sedating action on the brain, with some being more powerful than others. Such drugs can severely affect the awareness and performance level of the children taking them.

The aim of the doctor when beginning anti-convulsant treatment is to find the lowest possible drug level that will control the seizures without adversely affecting the awareness of the child. However, in a case where the epilepsy proves difficult to control, a higher level of medication may have to be used, or different drugs used in combination, often resulting in depressed brain function. In these situations, the desired aim of bringing the epilepsy under some sort of control may be achieved, but only at the cost of subjecting the child to the adverse effects of the drugs.

This may vary from just a mild level of drowsiness, to a significant degree of sedation. The effects are sometimes severe, and some children, as a result of taking high levels of medication, have trouble staying awake during the day. In extreme cases, where the level is very high, children literally sleep most of the day and night, a tragic situation indeed.

Fortunately, such severe effects are not observed in many brain injured children suffering from epilepsy, but a significant number are under some degree of sedation as a result of the medication they are taking. This can have an adverse effect on their development – they are already having difficulty functioning as a consequence of their brain injury, and this can be further aggravated by the effects of the medication. The sedation can act as another barrier between the environment and the brain thereby reducing the amount of sensory stimulation reaching the brain. It can also make motor function more difficult.

There appears to be a misunderstanding about the cause and effect relationship between brain injury and epilepsy. Many parents of children with epilepsy assume that most types of seizure can cause further brain injury; therefore, even though they may not like giving their child medication because of the side effects it can cause, they would prefer this to his brain being affected further by the seizures. The general attitude is that every attempt should be made to stop the seizures from occurring.

However, only in very severe cases are the seizures actually damaging to the brain or detrimental to the child. Dekaban[3] states: 'There is no doubt that *frequent* epileptic attacks occuring *daily* during early life will produce retardation of development, or even regression in a proportion of patients.' Dekaban reports that in the six children he studied, the frequency of seizures was high, averaging from eight to 100 a day. In extreme cases, a condition known as 'status epilepticus' may develop, with seizures occurring continuously without the patient regaining consciousness – this is potentially harmful to the brain. Also, a grand mal convulsion that causes the patient to stop breathing for a prolonged period may result in some injury to the brain due to a lack of oxygen.

But, these are the most extreme forms of epilepsy, and they only happen in a very small number of cases. They are the only instances where epilepsy can cause a decrease in function as a result of further brain injury. No one is really sure what happens in the brain at the time of a seizure. It is possible that the abnormal electrical activity destroys some brain cells, but this is not necessarily harmful. As we mentioned earlier in the book, normal people are continually losing brain cells without any loss of function, since the spare capacity of the brain can be utilized. The critical factor is the severity of the injury to the brain – if the epilepsy does destroy cells, but only to an insignificant degree, then no loss of function should occur. The proof that epilepsy is not necessarily harmful to the brain is the fact that most children who have seizures do not get worse, except when the seizures are of the severe kind mentioned earlier. If all seizures were harmful, you would expect the child to continually lose function.

Most types of epilepsy suffered by brain injured children do not adversely affect the function and health of the brain. Rather, it is the other way around, the brain injury causes the epilepsy – the epilepsy does not cause the brain injury.

Evidence that epilepsy is not necessarily harmful to the brain is demonstrated by the fact that many normal people suffer from mild forms of it without ever knowing. Walter Alvarez[4], a U.S.A. professor of medicine, describes many examples of what he calls nonconvulsive epilepsy. He says that many things like sleep walking, tossing in your sleep, headaches and nightmares may be the result of a very mild form of epilepsy. And yet, people with these symptoms lead normal lives, and there is no question of these seizure-like episodes causing brain injury.

As a consequence of the pervading fear of epilepsy, it is usually accepted that its control is the most important priority, and to achieve this end, a child may have to suffer the consequences of high levels of medication. But, just what price has to be paid to achieve this control? If the child is having severe or continual seizures, or if they are having a detrimental effect on his function, then an initial attempt must be made to suppress the seizures with medication. If the seizures are not severe and do not appear to be adversely affecting the child, then the question should be asked as to whether it would be appropriate to use medication. Is the control of a mild problem that is not harmful to the brain worth the possible detrimental effects of the medication?

It would be irresponsible to question the use of anti-convulsants without offering another way of approaching the problem. Before there can be any question of reducing or stopping the medication, an alternative means of bringing the seizures under control has to be found. Just stopping the drugs will not solve the problem, as the seizures will usually return or get worse. Instead, a way has to be found of treating the *cause* of the seizures.

One way this can be done is to put the child on an intensive neurological stimulation program based on the principles described in this book. If this treatment is successful in improving the function of the brain, there is a possibility that it will also decrease the epileptic activity in the brain – since this has been caused by the brain injury.

Other areas of treatment that should be looked at are nutrition and allergies. Some children's epilepsy has improved when they were placed on a high quality diet, and in some cases, seizures have been related to food and chemical allergies.

It is vitally important that in the initial stages of these alternative treatments, medication levels should *not* be touched. If the child responds, and the epilepsy decreases significantly, it may then be possible to consider a drug reduction. However, this should only be done in cooperation with the child's doctor, and it must be carried out *very* gradually.

If these approaches prove unsuccessful, it may be necessary to begin or continue the use of medication in an attempt to bring the seizures under control. However, if the child has a very mild form of epilepsy, with minor seizures occurring only a couple of times a month, or even less frequently, it may not be worth paying the price of possible side effects from the medication. The seizures do not adversely affect the child, but the medication might. But of course, each case has to looked at individually.

It is possible that some types of epilepsy can get worse when a child is exposed to certain types of stimulation used in therapy. However, this occurs in only a very small number of cases. If it does happen, the remedy is simple – the responsible activity needs to be modified or stopped completely. As long as this change in the therapy program is made soon after the increase in seizures is first observed, this increase should only be temporary.

We must reiterate that you should *not* stop giving your child medication just because you have begun an alternative treatment program. However, medication may be gradually decreased under a doctor's supervision, if the child makes significant progress.

It seems logical that, if the function of the brain can be improved through an intensive therapy program, epilepsy – a symptom of brain injury – can be decreased. If a child's speech, movement or eyesight can be improved by achieving better brain function, then it may also be possible to improve the epilepsy. In fact, this has been seen with some of the children treated in accordance with the methods described in this book. In most cases, the epilepsy of these children showed no sign of improvement before they commenced therapy, but they began to have fewer seizures as their function improved. It does not happen in all cases, and sometimes the seizures still persist. But the fact that some children have shown improvement is a good reason to consider it as a viable means of treatment.

Rather than just concentrating on one form of treatment, as is the situation today, it is best to consider anything that can possibly help – especially since the current approach is primarily symptomatic, is not always successful, and has potentially detrimental side-effects. As has been advocated all through this book, it is better to treat the cause of the problem, rather than the symptoms.

CHAPTER TWENTY-EIGHT

Discipline

IT IS not our intention in this chapter to tell a parent how to discipline a brain injured child, for this is for the parent to determine. Rather, we want to talk briefly about the *importance* of discipline.

Sometimes, the issue of discipline and brain injured children becomes similar to that of nutrition, and for the same reasons. Out of the extreme frustration of not knowing how they can best help their child, the parents' main aim is to make the child as happy as possible. As well, they naturally feel sorry for him, and they may think that it would not be fair to be too strict with him. Thus, he often gets away with being naughty, and he can break some of the rules that the other children in the family have to follow. Besides, his function is extremely limited, so isn't it best to encourage him to do whatever he can, even if it is not the right kind of behaviour?

All of these reactions are reasonable, given the situation the parents are in. However, there is a danger that if not disciplined properly the child will develop behavioural problems. The brain injured child has enough problems as it is, without any more being added to the list. To demonstrate our point, let us look at a couple of hypothetical examples using children who, although fictitious, are compilations of children and situations we have seen over the years.

* * *

'Susie' is four years old, but already she is in charge of her house. Her brain injury is primarily in the midbrain area, and as a result she has severe movement problems. Only now is she learning to get up on her hands and knees, and even that takes an enormous effort. However, her cortex seems to be working very well, for she is extremely bright. In fact, she seems to be as intelligent as most other four-year-olds. What's more she has very good speech, so much so that her parents jokingly complain that she never stops talking!

Being as clever as she is, she quickly understood the way that her parents felt about her. She realized that they were prepared to do almost anything for her, and all she needed to do was drop her bottom lip a little, or roll her beautiful brown eyes, and suddenly she would get what she wanted. It was even better when grandma and grandpa were around – why, they were a piece of cake!

Thus, Susie had developed her own set of rules about how to get what she wanted. All she had to do was ask for it, and if that didn't work, she could flash her pretty little eyes and use her endless charm. If all that failed, she could always resort to throwing a little tantrum, or a big one if necessary, for this nearly always succeeded.

Before her parents had realized what was happening, the whole dynamics of their house had changed, for the power structure had been turned upside down. Little Susie had become queen of the house. Nobody really could be blamed for this. It was not a weakness on behalf of the parents. She was so cute and loveable, and yet so helpless, so what else could they have done? It certainly wasn't Susie's fault, she had only made the best of a bad situation, without knowing any different. Children only learn the rules as they are presented to them.

Unfortunately, things started to get worse. By the time she had her fourth birthday, Susie's parents found it extremely difficult to get her to do anything that she didn't want to, without her throwing a tantrum. They were the ones following the commands, not her. It was worse when they went out anywhere because Susie knew that if she started to scream her parents would get embarrassed and give in to her almost immediately.

Around the same time, her parents were becoming very concerned with her mobility problems, as she was getting further and further behind her peers. They decided to begin an intensive home therapy program in an attempt to improve her function. However, Susie had other ideas. She was quite happy with her life just the way it was. She had everything she needed, and she could almost always get what she wanted, so she had nothing to complain about. Unlike her parents, she did not have the value of foresight. She couldn't see what it would be like if, ten years later, she was still unable to walk. Like all four-year-olds, all she was concerned about was the here and now, and as far as she could see everything was fine and dandy.

Naturally then, she saw the therapy program that her parents were trying to do with her as being an intrusion into her comfortable little world. Some of the exercises were fun, but others weren't. Anyway, it was much more enjoyable sitting on grandma's lap, or being taken for a walk in the stroller.

So, our indignant four-year-old decided to put a stop to the therapy. Every time anybody tried to do some work with her, she would let them know in no uncertain terms what she thought of it. She would scream and cry, and stiffen up so much that they couldn't even bend her legs. It became virtually impossible to do anything with her. As soon as they stopped trying to get her to work, she stopped crying and once again became cute and loveable. Thus, peace and sanity were restored – and so too was Susie's idea of who was in charge.

Her parents were exasperated, for they were only trying to do what they believed was best. But, as important as the therapy was, they simply could not do it. They had tried every approach, from cajoling to castigation, to no avail. Finally, they had no choice other than stopping the treatment program. They hoped that maybe they could try again in a couple of years time, when Susie was a little older and more understanding of what needed to be done. At the same time, they knew that they were running a risk, that without proper treatment her problems might get worse. But they could only hope that this wouldn't happen.

Discipline problems as severe as Susie's are rare in reality. Although some children like her may initially resist the treatment program, this is only to be expected since most people resist major changes in their lives. It is important in these early stages to persist and not give in to the child, for in most cases they will soon cooperate and actually enjoy the program. The success of this primarily depends on the parents' attitude. If you think that implementing the program is going to be impossible, the child is likely to sense this and the endeavour may fail.

* * *

'Ben' has just turned five, and his problems are very different to Susie's. He can walk and run, but he has very limited understanding and speech. Just as the problems of these two children are different, so too are the difficulties faced by their parents. Although Ben's parents can see that his comprehension and communication skills aren't developing as they should, they don't know what to do about it. Nor do they know how to discipline him, since his poor understanding makes this very difficult.

In the beginning, what concerned Ben's parents most was that he had no means of communicating his needs. As he got older, it seemed that he wanted to try and tell them something, but he just couldn't make himself understood. This was obviously very frustrating for all concerned, but his parents were overjoyed when they eventually discovered that at least some means of communication had been established. It seemed that every time Ben wanted something or needed to attract their attention, he would slap their arm. As soon as he did this, they would pick him up and praise him, while trying to determine what it was that he wanted.

Since his action was suitably rewarded, Ben quickly learnt this was a way of getting what he wanted, and thus he did it more and more. Unfortunately, at the age of five his speech had still not developed, and he still had to rely on non-verbal communication. He had established other ways of doing this apart from slapping, but this was still the most effective. But now this behaviour had developed into a problem, for he slaps people continually during the day, and it is often simply an attention-getting device. Also, he is now getting strong, and his slaps are beginning to hurt, especially when he does it to other children. Unfortunately, other parents think that Ben is an aggressive child and they are becoming reluctant to let their children play with him. What began as an innocent form of communication has now developed into socially unacceptable behaviour.

* * *

These are obviously two very different types of children with equally different discipline problems, but both situations have stemmed from the same cause – the absence of any real guidelines for the parents to follow as to how best to discipline their children. Susie and Ben are extreme examples, and it is not very often that children have problems that are so severe. However, there are degrees of Susie and Ben in many brain injured children.

The discipline problems of children like Susie are easier to deal with than those of children such as Ben. They are clever, and they understand from an early age what you are saying to them. The most important thing is that discipline needs to be established early, before the child tries to rearrange the power structure of the family.

As much as possible, they should be disciplined in exactly the same way as a normal child of the same age. Some people may think it unfair to do this to a child who has so many problems, but it is the best thing for both the parents and the child. If administered in a loving and caring way, discipline doesn't make a normal child unhappy, so why should it detract from the happiness of someone who is brain injured? Such children need special love and care, but they don't need to become king or queen of the house at the same time. Because they are so smart, children like Susie can understand a properly structured discipline program, and they usually respond very well to it as long as it is instituted early. Little children need guidelines to follow, and these need to be clearly defined and consistently reinforced – by both parents. Like all children, they will quickly learn to play off one parent against the other if the parents have different sets of rules.

Children like Ben present a completely different problem, for his lack of understanding prevents his comprehension of directions. But, even if he is unable to understand the word 'no', the parent may be able to convey the meaning of this word by a suitable tone of voice, or look of displeasure. Although simple, if this type of communication is applied consistently and appropriately, it may be the means of teaching him the basic rules of what he can and can't do. If parents can get this far, at least it will give them something to work on.

For such children, it is usually best to have everything very well structured, so as to make it easy for them to learn what's right and wrong. As frustrating as it may seem at the time, they respond best to constant repetition, so parents have to be very patient and constantly reinforce the simple rules that have been laid down. As well, somewhere along the way, a differentiation needs to be made between acceptable and unacceptable behaviour. As good as Ben's attempts at communication were, they eventually reached the point where they were socially unsuitable, so apart from trying to develop speech, simple but appropriate methods of communication need to be established.

Discipline is vitally important for brain injured children. Just like those who are normal, they need a clearly defined set of guidelines to follow. Without such structure, they may try and change the rules to their own advantage, as did Susie. Or, like Ben, they may develop anti-social behaviour, producing yet another problem that the parents have to deal with. If it is accepted that structure and discipline are important for normal children, then the same should apply to those who are brain injured.

Section VI
Is It Practical?

CHAPTER TWENTY-NINE

Parents as Therapists

DOES the suggestion that parents of brain injured children become the primary therapists for their children, threaten a demarcation dispute? Should therapy only be carried out by properly trained therapists, or can it be done by the parents with the therapist taking on a supervisory role?

Before these questions can be answered, it has to be realized that, no matter how well trained a therapist may be, there is one advantage that parents will always possess. As parents, they usually have more dedication and motivation to do all they can for their child, and they are often willing and able to give the individual attention that is required. Furthermore, they know and understand the child better than anyone else and, as a result, can usually get the best performance out of the child.

These are attributes that a therapist can never have, and yet they are vital to a successful treatment program. So what if the two were combined – *the therapist's technical knowledge and practical experience* with *the parents' understanding and love of their child*? Surely this would be the best way in which to conduct a treatment program.

The parents cannot teach the therapist how to be the mother or father of their child, but the therapist can show the parents how to carry out the treatment required, providing that the techniques to be used are not too complicated. In this way, the talents of those involved would be utilized to the fullest – the therapist would devise and update the appropriate treatment program, and this would then be administered by the parents. In such a situation, parents have repeatedly demonstrated that they can make excellent therapists for their child. Parents possess a tremendous raw material – the love they have for their child – and this needs to be taken advantage of. Many parents are certainly willing to get directly involved in the treatment. In fact, parents often find that one of the most overwhelming aspects of having a brain injured child is that feeling of helplessness through not knowing what to do about their child's lack of progress.

This raw material needs to be refined and channelled in the right direction, a process that requires several steps. First of all, the nature of their child's brain injury needs to be fully explained to them. After the child has been assessed, someone needs to sit down with them and carefully go over the results of the evaluation. If a measuring tool such as the Sandler-Brown Developmental Profile is used, it is possible to present this information clearly and concisely. Once the parents realize what sort of problems their child has, they begin to understand why he can't do the things that he should be doing.

The next step in the refinement process is to teach the parents about the brain – how it works and how it can be treated. The better they understand the nature of the brain, the better therapists they will become. Here, as with most things in life, the more you know about what you are doing, the easier the task becomes. This teaching cannot be done in half an hour, given the complexity of the subject matter. Instead, it requires at least six to eight hours of intensive instruction.

The final step involves teaching the treatment program to the parents, a program that is carefully designed in accordance with each child's specific problems. Since the type of treatment advocated in this book is based on the principles of normal development, all of the treatment techniques are easy to administer. Nature does not need fancy equipment to ensure that normal babies develop correctly, just lots of stimulation, opportunity and love. And so it is with this particular method of treatment. All the techniques are designed so they can be easily performed by parents.

Since the treatment program has to be applied with the correct frequency, intensity and duration, the parents are the only people who are in a position to spend the time that is required with the child. It would be uneconomical for a therapist to spend all his time with one patient, and virtually impossible for a child to receive such individual care in an institutional setting. This does not mean that all parents of brain injured children should be forced to administer the treatment program to their child. For some, this would be impossible. However, there are parents who choose to become completely involved, and it is for these parents that an intensive, home-based treatment program is offered.

Although some people may think it unfair to expect parents to carry out their own therapy program, it is interesting to note that this opportunity for complete involvement is one of the main aspects that attracts parents to this type of treatment. Many have been desperately looking for something 'to get their teeth into', for they usually realize very quickly that there are not going to be any easy answers. They know that if their child is going to improve, it will require lots of hard work on their behalf. Even if the child doesn't respond as much as they would have liked, at least they will know that they have done all they can to help him.

Another important aspect of a parent-run treatment program is that it can be carried out in the home environment. The familiar surroundings of home are reassuring to most brain injured children. In an unfamiliar environment, the child may feel threatened and afraid. Taking him to a therapy centre, no matter how pleasant the place may be, can make the child tense and upset, and in such a state he is unlikely to perform at his best for the therapist. And, no matter how nice the therapist is, he or she is *not* mummy or daddy. A severely brain injured child is completely dependent on his mother, and to take him away from his lifeline and place him in a strange environment with many unfamiliar people may be an extremely traumatic experience.

It seems to be human nature that most people work better if everything is well structured and highly organized. It is a rare person who can work to maximum output without some sort of external control. This applies as much to parents of brain injured children as it does to anyone else. Many parents complain that when they go to a therapy centre, they are often not told exactly what has to be done with their child on a daily basis. They may be shown treatment techniques they can carry out at home, but the instructions they receive are usually vague. They may be told to do the exercises when both they and their child are in the mood, or to fit them in between all the other things that need to be done around the house. They are never really told exactly when they should be done, or how many times they should be repeated.

Thus, without a specific timetable, the parents, being no different to most of us, tend to put off what needs to be done. There are always other things that need their attention. Since no one stresses to them the importance of constant repetition, the therapy is usually performed in a rather spasmodic way. Although the parents often feel that this is not right, they find it difficult to correct their ways since they have no clear guidelines to follow.

If a home-based therapy program is to be successful, the parents need to know *exactly* what they are required to do on a day-to-day basis. Thus, everything should be clearly set out and organized in such a way that the parents have a specific daily timetable to follow. Of course, there will be days when, for whatever reason, it will not be possible to carry out the full quota of what is required, but at least it will be clear what should be attempted each day.

* * *

Angelina Perroni of Perth, Western Australia, carried out an intensive home treatment program for two and a half years with her daughter Pia. Her following comments clearly demonstrate the need for a properly organized treatment program:

For two long years I had been constantly searching for medical help for my daughter who has a problem known as 'Noonan's Syndrome' (a genetic abnormality). I had only been offered minimal support from the orthodox medical establishments, so the idea of a treatment program that I could carry out myself was very attractive. Before I began this type of treatment, any therapy I had done was based on my own initiative and instincts, and was performed on a part-time basis. I knew that this was not enough to get her well, and I sensed that she was capable of much more. I also discovered what a lonely and frustrating world it is when a mother doesn't know just how best she can help her child.

When I embarked on the home treatment program, I was grateful for two reasons. It meant that I would finally be working in an organized manner, and since it was a task I could not perform alone, I knew that there was a good chance that I would be able to receive assistance from the community in the form of volunteer help.

Having been a university tutor prior to the birth of my children, I was very aware of the need to be properly organized, and to work to a specific time schedule. Therefore, I was elated when I was presented with a therapy program that relied heavily on organization and running to time. Here was someone setting out my day's work – all I had to do was make sure that it was carried out. It was almost as if someone had done all the research work on a thesis, and all I had to do was write it up. No more wondering what to do with Pia, no more questioning about whether what I was doing was right, no more doubting myself or my child. It was simply a matter of getting on with the job.

However, before I could effectively do what was required, I had to first understand the reason behind what I was going to do. The many hours of lectures not only helped me understand Pia's problems better, but I also learn about the functions of the brain, and about child development, nutrition and behaviour. In fact, I learnt more about my child during the three days of the initial evaluation than I had in the two years of her entire life. This, combined with the training of how to carry out the therapy at home, meant that I felt in complete control of the situation for the first time since Pia was born. I was now well equipped mentally and pyschologically to carry out a task which had previously seemed impossible – to try and make my child better.

What had before appeared to be such a daunting prospect now became a challenge. I had taken on a new role – that of parent-therapist. I, solely, would be responsible for the smooth running of the program. But at the same time, I hoped that I would receive help in carrying it out by way of volunteers. It was reassuring to know that I no longer had to battle along by myself.

One of the criticisms that is sometimes made of a parent-based treatment program is that it often has a detrimental effect on the family, particularly the husband-wife relationship. It is true such a program is not easy to carry out, as there is usually quite a deal of work to be done, but this does not automatically mean that it is bad for the family structure.

It must be realized that just having a brain injured child undoubtedly puts pressure on any family. The doubt, the uncertainty, the apparently bleak future for the child, are all things that the family has to cope with. In some cases, marriages have broken up as an apparent result of the presence of a brain injured child in the family.

Sherry Wright[1], a Brisbane marriage and relationship counsellor, conducted a survey to investigate the effect that a brain injured child has on the family. Fifty-two parents responded to the question: 'What effect does a disabled child have on your family relationships?'. Of these, twenty-nine (56 per cent) said that it had a major negative effect, eight (15 per cent) reported a minimal negative effect, nine (17 per cent) said there was no effect, and three (6 per cent) said it had a positive effect. Although the number of parents surveyed was small, these statistics give a valuable guide to just how much the presence of a brain injured child can disrupt the family.

At the same time as this Brisbane survey, the Australian Centre for Brain Injured Children decided to investigate what effects a home-based treatment program had on the families involved. As part of the survey that was mentioned in the Introduction (Appendix 1), one of the questions asked was: 'How did the intensity of the treatment program affect your family?'

The parents were asked to select one of the following answers:

1. There were major family problems
2. There were mild family problems
3. No effect, either adverse or positive
4. Positive effect on family unit

If an intensive, home-based treatment program is as bad for family relationships as some people claim it to be, it would be expected that the vast majority of parents would have indicated that it had created a major family problem – especially when it was found in the Brisbane survey that 56 per cent of the parents indicated that just having a brain injured child, *without* the added burden of carrying out a treatment program, had a major negative effect. However, of the 146 parents who responded to the question, only *twelve (8 per cent)* said that the treatment program caused major family problems. Sixty-one (42 per cent) said that it resulted in minor family problems, and 16 (11 per cent) said it had no effect, positive or negative.

Most people would not think that having a brain injured child would be a positive influence on the family, and this is borne out by the fact that only 6 per cent of the parents involved in the Brisbane survey indicated that this was the case. The most startling fact about the survey of the parents involved in treating their children at home, was that *fifty-seven (39 per cent)* said that this, in fact, had a positive effect on their family relationships. No one has ever discussed the possible positive effects of home-based treatment programs before, as all attention has been directed at the possible harmful effects. It is worthwhile looking at some of the positive comments made by parents on their returned questionnaires:

It gave us a common goal, and educated the public a great deal.

Our other son suffered no ill-effects, in fact he is now very proud of what his brother has achieved.

People always say that a program of this kind will destroy a family, but if anything, we have never been as close as we are now.

We had a happier family unit because we were giving our son all we could in every way, and that meant contentment.

We all shared in the program and felt that it was a special year of giving and loving, despite the intensity of commitment required.

It is of obvious concern that 50 per cent of the families surveyed did suffer some adverse effects, but this is inevitable when dealing with a problem that, therapy or no therapy, puts a strain on any family. This points to the need for greater social and government support for such families, both in coping with the child and his disabilities, and with carrying out a treatment program, if this is what the parents choose to do.

But, it is important to note that there can be *positive* effects on the family unit as a result of a home therapy program. We do not say that all families should be involved with therapy if one of their members is brain injured, as this is an individual choice for those concerned. However, it is important to realize that some families can cope very well with such a program, so why should they be denied the opportunity to work with their child because of the general assumption that an intense home program adversely affects the family?

It is also often said that the other children in the family will automatically suffer if home therapy is instituted. But, often the brothers and sisters get involved with the treatment – not because they are made to, but because they want to do all they can to help. Just like their parents, they too have been frustrated at not knowing what they could do.

If the siblings are too young to comprehend this, they often get involved simply because to them lots of things in the treatment program are just good fun – like rolling around or creeping on their hands and knees around the house, chasing after, or being chased by, their brother or sister.

Perhaps the words of Chrissy Adams of Minnesota, U.S.A., best describe the attitude often seen in older brothers and sisters:

My name is Chrissy and I'm twelve. My sister Anya is brain injured. She's two-and-a-half.

When I found out that my sister was retarded, it was scary. I felt like I could only tell my best friends, and when I did they sort of ignored me for a while. But when Anya started the program, I wanted to tell them all about it. Without having to try hardly at all, we got a speech together, and it was fun giving it to the whole sixth grade. Some of them even came to help.

Working with her is real fun. Even though we have bad days, it is still fun. When I go away for a week or even a few days, you can see changes in her.

Our family has gotten closer as time goes on, and in that way it doesn't seem so bad. I have had lots of changes in myself too, like I can relate better to Anya than I could have if I didn't work with her on the program.

All in all, I feel that her being on the program is not a burden, but an experience.

CHAPTER THIRTY

A Community Responsibility

ALTHOUGH this book advocates a parent-run treatment program, the onus of its administration should not fall on the parents alone. It takes tremendous courage on their behalf to take on such a challenge, and since they often have to go against their doctor's advice, they receive very little support from professional people. If they are to succeed, they need support from the community in lots of different ways.

The most direct assistance they require is in the form of volunteer help to carry out the treatment program. They often have other children to take care of along with other responsibilities that have to be met, so it may be difficult for them to run the program without any outside help. In some cases, parents have chosen to carry it out alone and have managed quite successfully, but in most situations, physical support is necessary.

This system of utilizing volunteer help usually works very well. Since the treatment program described in this book is designed so that it can be administered by parents and helpers, no special qualifications are needed. Many of the volunteers comment on how simple the therapy is to do. The only attributes that are needed are some spare time, and plenty of love.

Most parents are concerned when first confronted with the prospect of trying to find people to come in and help them. This is especially true of those who live in a city. They may not even know the people in the neighbourhood, let alone be friendly enough to ask them for their help. It is usually easier to recruit volunteers in country areas, given the strong community spirit that exists in most country towns. But, even in the city, parents are often amazed at the many offers of help that come in when word of their need spreads. People whom they have never met before are suddenly willing to devote some of their time to come and help a child in need.

A family living in a rural area of Western Australia were dumb-struck at the response they received to their appeal for help. Over one hundred people offered to work with their child. There were so many that each person was only required once every two weeks. And it was not just local people who volunteered their services – some came from up to fifty kilometres away, and they complained that they were not needed weekly!

It's no wonder that many of the parents report that the response they receive goes a long way to restoring their faith in human nature. Every time you pick up a newspaper it seems that all you read about are the bad things going on in the world, so it's refresh-ing to see so many people rallying to help a child and his parents. As well, it's nice to know that in our increasingly mechanized society, where people's services are becoming more and more redundant, there is something that relies solely on human-power. No machine can ever take the place of the volunteers.

Another way that the community can be of assistance to parents of brain injured children is in the formation of self-help support groups. In Australia, there is a network of support groups known as 'Friends of Brain Injured Children'. These groups have been extre-mely successful in achieving their aims. In most cases, they are not parents of brain injured children themselves, but simply members of the community with a strong desire to help. They provide sup-port by assisting the parents in organizing the program, arranging for volunteers, helping in the construction and distribution of equip-ment that may be needed, and, in some cases, organizing fund raising activities. In general, they give the parents lots of moral support and a welcome helping hand.

The utilization of community resources in the treatment of brain injured children greatly benefits all three parties concerned, and this benefit is sometimes derived in unexpected ways. The most obvious people to benefit are the parents. As we mentioned before, in many cases they would not be able to carry out the therapy without assistance. But they receive much more than just physical support. Many parents have to deal with the enormous problems of caring for a brain injured child on their own, for there are few people to whom they can turn for support. Often it seems to them that they are fighting a lone battle. Thus, their spirit and strength is lifted enormously at the sight of complete strangers coming into their house, full of love and concern for their child. What's more, these volunteers ask for nothing in return.

Angelina Perroni, the Western Australian parent whose comments were given in the previous chapter, describes here her reactions to all the help that she received when she was working with her daughter:

While many professionals may argue that volunteers are an intrusion into people's privacy, I welcomed them with open arms. They gave me physical, emotional and psychological support throughout the two-and-a-half years we were on the program. Without them, I could not have even considered undertaking a home treatment program. To this day it still amazes me how so many people rallied to the support of someone in need.

As well as assisting me physically in doing the therapy, the volunteers also helped in many other ways. For instance, they were an endles source of ideas for stimulating and encouraging Pia to do her work. They often offered to make aids for the program, such as reading cards, pictures and numbers. They brought with them toys that they thought Pia would be interested in. They even offered to do work other than with the program, such as child minding and ironing, or they simply took over the workroom so that I could get away for a while.

They were not only a great help to me, for they also greatly contributed to Pia's progress. They were a great source of social interaction for her. This occurred outside as well as inside the workroom, for they often took her for walks, on outings, or invited her to play with their siblings. The constant love and encouragement showered on Pia by the volunteers helped to mould her into a confident, affable, loving child.

They were also useful in keeping Pia's progress in perspective. Being so close to her, I often didn't notice the many little ways she was changing. But, as they were only seeing her once a week, they often noticed how she was improving – little things that I had overlooked. Thus, I found their comments to be a constant source of encouragement.

The volunteers were my lifeline, and I will be forever grateful to those generous and loving people who helped our daughter walk, talk, and grow in every sense of the word.

As can be seen from Angelina's comments, the child also benefits greatly from having people coming in to carry out the therapy. Although the situation has improved lately, most brain injured children never get a chance to be part of normal society. They go off to special schools or therapy centres on special buses, and rarely mix with normal people. Except for their own brothers and sisters and relations, many brain injured children miss out on a great deal of normal social interaction with both children and adults.

A home-based therapy program changes all of that for, suddenly, the child becomes the centre of attention. All of the people are coming in to his home just to be with him. It must be a tremendous psychological boost for the child to be the recipient of so much love and concern. As well, the volunteers often bring their own children with them, so this ensures that the child on the program gets the opportunity to be with normal children, even while he is working.

The volunteers often get a great deal of pleasure, satisfaction and fulfilment from their involvement with the treatment program. When they begin, many are nervous and unsure about what to expect, especially if they have not had any previous experience with brain injured children. However, they quickly discover that the child simply needs lots of love and attention, just like other children. They also gain great joy from seeing the child progress, and even the smallest sign of improvement causes great excitement. Many of the volunteers become much more than just people paying a weekly visit, for they become completely involved in the child's development. Often, after their child is reassessed, parents are besieged by helpers telephoning to see how the child went.

Here is how some volunteers describe their experience of working with a child. Anne Harrison of Sydney writes:

I have been working with Carlo since he first went on to the program. I must admit that when I saw him for the first time, I wondered how we would ever be able to get him mobile, for he could only roll from side to side. However, it soon became obvious that he had tremendous determination and willpower, and this was helpful for what had to be achieved.

I think that Carlo and children like him teach us all a great lesson in humility, courage, determination and faith. He has made me aware that brain injured children are God's special people to be loved just as everyone else. I have learned to see these children through new eyes, and can now relate to handicapped people with much more ease.

Phyllis Brevig, of Minnesota, U.S.A.:

Have you ever had the thrill of hearing a child say her first sentence? I have! I will never forget when Jesse said: 'Get your nose'. Each week I see new improvements, and if I never accomplish anything else in my life, I know I will always have the thrill of remembering Jesse's progress to a normal and productive life. If 'normal' adults had her patience and determination, we would have a land of giants!

Peggy Frank Keenan, also of Minnesota:

The sign on the bulletin board at the neighbourhood grocery store said a family was looking for volunteers to work with their two-and-a-half-year-old brain injured daughter, Anya. When I first met Anya, I was reminded of a Raggedy-Anne doll, as her arms and legs hung loosely at her sides, unable to be used in a purposeful way. Her muscle tone was poor, and she was unable to crawl or creep – although she could sit up by herself, but even then she was very shaky. In lots of ways she was very much like a newborn infant.

During our first session together, I learnt to work her daily routine consisting of a series of tasks or exercises. Anya made it clear that it was as new to her as it was to me, and she was obviously upset about what was going on. However, we carried on despite the continual crying, and as the weeks passed, the cries were soon replaced with giggles as she became used to the exercises and all the different people working with her.

I have been excited to see progress in all areas of her development during the past few months. She has gained considerable strength and weight, and she now crawls through the house with great independance. I hear lots of vocalizations now, and will not be surprised if I hear a distinguishable word soon.

Jeff and Linda Haefemeyer, Minnesota:

We had never worked with a handicapped child before, and were uncertain about our ability to help Anya. After working with her, these apprehensions soon went away. It has been a growing and enriching experience for us, as well as a satisfying one.

CHAPTER THIRTY-ONE

You and Your Doctor

U NTIL now, a doctor has had very few options available as to what he can offer the parents of brain injured children. If the child is cerebral palsied, he can suggest the local spastic centre; if the child is autistic, then there is the autistic school; for those who are mentally retarded, there is always the local special school. Apart from telling parents that they can always keep their child at home, a doctor can't really offer the parents a choice of where their child could be treated. Although the conventional treatment centres and schools established for brain injured children do some good work, the absence of any alternatives is a far from satisfactory situation.

Since parents are usually given little encouragement to keep the child at home and become involved in an intensive home therapy program, they have little choice other than to send their child to an appropriate therapy centre or school. Even if they are subsequently unhappy with the treatment their child is receiving, they have no real alternatives to consider.

If parents of brain injured children are unsatisfied with the choice of treatment that has been suggested for their child, or if after their child has received this treatment they are not happy with his progress, one of the people to whom they may turn for advice is the family doctor. He may be familiar with their child, since many brain injured children are frequently in and out of doctors' rooms. Also, being the family doctor, he may be aware of the dynamics of the whole family, and how it copes with the stresses and strains of having a brain injured child.

If you, as a parent, are interested in any type of alternative therapy for your child, you may want to seek a medical opinion of the particular treatment you are considering, and you may indeed consult your family doctor. If you don't have one, or you are not happy with your present one, it would be best to try and find a doctor with an open mind and a special interest in brain injured children.

But you should be very careful about the way in which you approach the doctor for advice. Depending on his attitude (which you may not know beforehand), it could be a delicate issue that needs to be handled correctly.

By considering an alternative means of therapy, you may find yourself in conflict with your doctor and with the existing medical system. The decision you have to make will be even more difficult if it means going against the advice of some professionals. It is our endeavour to show you how to make such a decision, while still trying to maintain a good patient-doctor relationship.

If you were officially informed that your child was brain injured, you may have also been told that it was a difficult problem to treat, and improvement would be slow and most probably limited. It is likely that you were presented with three opinions to consider, as these three options constitute the basic orthodox medical approach to brain injury.

You may have been told that the best thing to do was to adopt what can best be described as the 'wait and see' approach. This is especially the case with very young children, since there is the chance that improvement may occur as a result of natural growth. Rather than actively intervening, this approach involves letting nature take its course, in the hope that your child will gradually improve.

Or, a more active option may have been presented – the suggestion of a therapy program designed to try and improve your child. Depending on the exact nature of your child's problems, this therapy probably would involve some form of speech therapy and/or occupational therapy and/or physiotherapy. Wanting to do as much as you can for your child, you may be a little surprised to discover that such treatment is offered in small doses – perhaps a weekly visit to the therapy centre, along with a small amount of therapy to be carried out at home.

The final option that may have been offered would, if adopted, have the most drastic effects on your child. It usually is applied only to severely brain injured children because such children are often thought to have no chance of recovery. In these circumstances, you may have been told that nothing could be done for your child and that the best thing for all concerned would be to put him into an institution. Often, no other choices are given, and such drastic action is taken simply because it seems that nothing else can be done.

It is natural for parents to want the best for their child, and to want to do everything possible to help him reach his full potential. If the child is normal, this potential is a rather nebulous thing, since how far the child eventually develops is dependent on many factors outside the control of parents. But for parents of brain injured children, the goal they have for their child is much more definable, for all they want is for him to be normal, or as near to normal as possible. To parents of normal children, this may seem a simple and reasonable request – something they take for granted. What they usually want is for their child to be better than normal.

Simple and reasonable as wanting a normal life for your child may sound, it is not so if your child is severely brain injured. For such parents, this goal often causes feelings of doubt and insecurity as over and over they ask themselves such questions as: 'Shouldn't we be satisfied with what we have got?' 'Aren't we just clutching at straws?' 'Maybe it was God's will, so who are we to want or demand more?'

Confronted by the three options that conventional medicine usually presents, such hopes for having a normal or near-normal child seem unrealistic and unreasonable. Parents are often told that the child will always have problems, and therefore it is something that just has to be accepted. They quickly become aware that the chances of their child making significant improvement with the 'wait and see' or 'there's nothing we can do' approaches are fairly remote. They may be given to understand that there is a good chance that the child will improve with the active intervention approach, but the amount of progress will be limited if such therapy is only given in small amounts.

Thus for these parents faced with the harsh realities of the world of brain injury, the desire for the child to be as close to normal as possible soon seems like an intangible dream. With the gradual demise of the parents' expectations goes the light of hope. Soon, the way ahead seems dark and never ending, the only relief coming with the acceptance that the child will never be normal.

Is this the way that it should be? Is it unrealistic and irrational for parents of a brain injured child to wish for significant and meaningful progress? If it could be shown that none of these children make any progress, then this would be so. But, the results of organizations such as the Australian Centre for Brain Injured Children suggest otherwise. They show, without making any promises, that some brain injured children can progress very well.

Those parents investigating alternative forms of therapy naturally do so hopeful that their child *will* advance beyond his present level. But when they go along to their doctor to seek his advice, how does he view their optimistic attitude and interest in something new?

First, it is necessary to understand the way the doctor may be looking at the problem. He has been taught to listen to his patients – to listen to their story, but constantly to weigh up what they are saying. He is trained to ask himself as he listens: 'is it reasonable; could it be true; is there an alternative to what I am being told?' 'Have a "high index of suspicion" ' is one of the rules he must live by. Every doctor has seen the girl who said that she 'couldn't possibly be pregnant' deliver at the appropriate time. Every doctor has smelt alcohol on the breath of the patient who swears he never drinks, or tobacco on the patient who says he has given up smoking. He has probably been misled and embarrassed in this way many times, and as a result he is wary of what he is told.

This critical attitude is also applied to his assessment of any treatment which is different from those taught in medical school, or described in medical journals. In this regard, he has been schooled: 'Never be the first to try the new, or the last to leave the old'. If he continues to follow the same principles as his colleagues, he can successfully remain part of mainstream medicine.

Given these considerations, how does a doctor usually view the problems of a brain injured child? Rather than hope, he may offer the parents sympathy, as he sees it as a problem without a solution. He would like to have something positive to offer, but his entire training and experience has shown him the catastrophe of brain injury. He knows that the conventional treatment of brain injury is one of the most difficult and unsuccessful areas of medicine. The results of orthodox treatment certainly support him in this conclusion.

He also knows the great strain that having a brain injured child places on a marriage, and on the other children in the family. He has seen or heard of marriages that have broken up as a result of this strain, or where the parents have tried to do too much and, having

failed to achieve what they wanted, have blamed each other. He has
seen the brothers and sisters of brain injured children feel separated and neglected by their parents. He naturally wants to reduce
the possibility of this happening to any family that he deals with.

He also feels that he should guard the parents against the im-
postor, the charlatan, the racketeer. He thinks that desperate
parents searching for any solution to help their child can be easily
taken advantage of with promises of hope and glory.

This is the background into which the idea of alternative therapy
is introduced. Therefore, if you simply tell the doctor that you want
to begin a particular method of treatment with your child, he is
likely to react in a negative way. He will most probably consider
that you are ignorant of this highly specialized area of medicine,
since you are *only* a parent, and that you are not properly informed
to make a rational judgement. The choice that you have made may
be contrary to his opinion, and he may see this as a challenge to his
competence. He will obviously question the authority of any people
who claim that something better can be done for brain injured
children, and will want to see evidence to back up their claims. He
may have previously warned you to stay away from such offers of
hope, and your decision would indicate to him that you have taken
no notice of his advice.

Instead of directly confronting your doctor, you should carefully
plan your approach if you want to get both an objective opinion and
his support for what you eventually decide to do.

Firstly, make a special appointment to see him. The discussion of
the treatment you are considering should be the only purpose of
this visit. Also, arrange a longer appointment than normal – your
doctor is probably quite busy, and he won't have the time to discuss
your proposal unless you make these special arrangements.

At this first appointment, simply ask for his advice. Tell him that
you have heard about a particular type of treatment, and you want
to explore the possibility of it helping your child. You probably will
not have made up your own mind at this stage, so you will appreciate any guidance he may be able to offer. But, you should tell him
that you do not want his opinion right away. His comments at this
first visit may be clouded by his emotional reaction to your suggestion, no matter how carefully you approach the subject, so do not
let him discuss it there and then. Instead, tell him that you would
like him to research this type of treatment and give it some careful

thought. Give him some information, preferably written and as concise as possible, and ask him to look through this for you. As well, ask him if he has any literature on the subject, and if so, if he could review this along with your material. If he dismisses your proposal out of hand, ask him if he would be prepared to look through your literature anyway. Tell him that you will make an appointment for three or four days later, so that he knows he has this time to read the literature and consider your proposal.

You must understand from the outset that there is very little chance that you, as a parent, are going to convince the doctor that you are 'right' and he is 'wrong'. Nor should you attempt to do so. This is not the time to be trying to win a battle – this is the opening discussion, and you cannot expect him to immediately agree with something that is probably new to him. At this point in time, all you are after is his advice and assistance in your decision making.

This is as far as you should go at the first appointment. Ask him when would be the best time for you to come back and discuss the matter in more depth, but do not let it go for longer than a week, otherwise it may slip his mind. When you make the next appointment with his receptionist, make a special point of asking her to let the doctor know the day when you will be returning.

In this interim period, you should do some homework yourself. Study carefully the literature you have on the subject. As well, try and make contact with other parents who have been carrying out this type of treatment, as your decision should not be based on just your doctor's opinion. Try and get as many viewpoints as you can. If possible, try and get the name of another doctor, one who has a positive attitude to the treatment of brain injured children, as you may like your doctor to consult with him – perhaps the parents you make contact with could help you with this.

When you return for your next visit, which like the first should be an extended one, you will be well prepared to discuss all the relevant issues. Both parents should attend, as this will show the doctor that they are working together. Do not be too disappointed if the doctor has not read any of the literature that you gave him. Give him the benefit of the doubt, as it may simply be because he was too busy. Make another appointment for two or three days later. In this situation, it is best to terminate the appointment there and then, otherwise the doctor may give his opinion without having properly researched the matter. He may have only looked at the critical articles, which would naturally give him a biased opinion. So it would be best to ask at the outset if he has read *all* of your material.

If your doctor has not read the information you gave him by the time you go back for your third visit, you should ask him directly if he is prepared to read the literature. If he is not, it doesn't automatically mean that he is opposed to you trying the therapy program, so you should ask him if he is opposed. If he says that he *is* against it, you should dismiss his advice and consult with someone else, since his opinion is not based on proper research.

If he is opposed to the idea, ask him why, and request that he backs up his opinions. If he quotes references that you have not seen, ask if he could either give you a copy of these, or at least explain them to you. Here you need to be forthright, but not rude or aggressive. Understand that this can be an emotional issue which sometimes affects people's judgements. You have a right as a patient to get as much information as you can from your doctor and, at the same time, you are quite justified in making sure that the advice being offered is correct. You should then ask him to listen to your side of the story – the reasons why you are considering the type of treatment being discussed.

If at the end of this appointment you find that the doctor is still opposed to the idea, then you have to respect his opinion, and also seriously consider his arguments. But you should not let one person's opinion be your only guide. You should tell your doctor that you intend to seek a second opinion. It is imperative that you do this independently of your doctor, as he may refer you to someone with similar views to his own. Remember that you can seek a second opinion from any doctor by yourself, without referral. As well, you should ask the doctor's secretary for a copy of all the relevant medical notes concerning your child, as the new doctor will need to see these. Do not take 'no' for an answer, as you have a right to demand that they either give the notes to you, or forward them directly to the doctor you are going to see.

Of course, if the doctor has read all the material and agrees with you to at least give it a try, this will help you make your decision. If you do choose to start the therapy program, tell your doctor that you would like him to look after the medical aspects of your child's problem, as well as monitoring the progress that hopefully will be made.

In the end, even if your doctor disagrees, you may still decide to try this alternative approach to your child's problem. You may make this decision for several reasons:

● You may think that the doctor has not been rational in his judgement.

● Despite what the doctor has said, you have read about or seen other children who have progressed as a result of this type of treatment, so you would like to see if it works for your child.

● You may decide that what orthodox medicine offers is not appropriate, and this type of therapy seems to be a much better approach to the problem.

While we would encourage you to obtain it, you don't need your doctor's approval to undergo the type of therapy advocated in this book. The role of the medical doctor in the management of brain injured children is twofold:

(1) He looks after the medical aspects of the problem, dealing with all the childhood illnesses that the child may encounter, and he plays a part in deciding on the most suitable therapeutic approach to the child's problem, and

(2) he recommends that the child should go to the spastic centre, or wherever.

But, a doctor *does not* get involved in the therapy side of the treatment, for this is the responsibility of therapists and parents. Therapy is not usually one of his specialities, and it is quite likely that he knows very little about this subject. All of this should be considered when you ask for your doctor's opinion on what is basically a question of therapy.

It is still quite possible to use the services of your doctor even if he is opposed to the therapy program. As long as he is willing to look after your child's health problems, then this is all you really need from him. Parents who have been in this situation have said that when they see the doctor, the therapy program is never mentioned. It would obviously be best to find a doctor who was supportive of your actions, but if you are perfectly happy with the *medical* service your doctor provides, it may just be a case of having to bite your tongue when you go to see him.

Special note for parents of children in coma

If your child is in coma, time is of the essence – you must act quickly. As we have already said, the longer a child remains in coma, the more difficult it usually is to arouse him, and the greater the chance of problems persisting once he regains consciousness.

Seeing that the child is still likely to be in hospital or a nursing home, you will need to get the permission of the doctors and administrators before you can begin a coma arousal program. Your approach should be similar to the one described in this chapter – make a special appointment to see the doctor, and present him with information about the coma arousal method, perhaps the relevant chapters from this book. Give him a day or two to read this, and then ask for his opinion.

Unless the doctor can present a very good reason for not instigating the coma arousal program, you should not be prepared to take 'no' for an answer. Be emphatic with the doctor – tell him that you are by your child's side most of the time anyway (as is often the case), so it will not take up any extra time. And tell him that at least you will feel that you are doing something positive and constructive for your child, rather than just helplessly watching him lie there. Impress upon him that there is nothing potentially harmful about the treatment, and anyway, his condition is constantly monitored by the hospital staff.

If the doctor is still opposed to or unsure of your request, ask him to at least consider a trial period, say for one month. At the end of this time, you and he can sit down and assess the results of your efforts to see if there has been any progress, and if this progress warrants you continuing the arousal program.

This issue is such a critical one that you should not settle with juust one doctor's opinion. Insist on at least one other doctor, if not more, looking at your child and considering your request to start working with him. If you find that all the medical staff are antagonistic to the concept of coma arousal, you should get an outside opinion – arrange for a doctor who is not employed at the hospital to come and look at your child. If possible, try and find someone who is at least aware of the principles of coma arousal. You will have to arrange this action through either your doctor or the medical superintendent of the hospital.

Be prepared to exert your rights as a parent of a patient in that hospital, for there is a lot at stake.

CHAPTER THIRTY-TWO

Your Doctor and You
By a General Practitioner

The medical doctor who has contributed this important chapter to the book is a general practitioner in a rural area of Western Australia. Here he describes, from the doctor's point of view, what it's like to be confronted by parents of a brain injured child who are wanting to try an alternative form of treatment. His frank comments provide valuable insight for both parents and doctors.

I had been in general practice for five years when I first encountered the question of alternative treatment for brain injured children. Up until this time, my approach to medicine had naturally been strongly influenced by my training. Like most medical students, I had been taught in a didactic rather than deductive way. The didactic method involves listening, learning and repeating exactly what is taught, until an authority greater than your teacher tells you otherwise. In contrast, the deductive approach involves observing what is taught and demonstrated, drawing your own conclusions, and then putting this knowledge into practice, while at all times maintaining an attitude of critical observation. Prior to my encounter with my brain injured patient, only a few fortunate experiences with enlightened specialists and highly educated patients had caused me to question my previous didactic training.

A severely brain injured child had been born in our area and was under the care of other doctors. I heard of this case, and had enormous sympathy for the parents and medical staff concerned, as I thought that very little could be done to help the child. My original anatomical and physiological training had firmly stated that central nervous system tissue never regenerated, therefore injury to the brain was most likely to result in a permanent loss of function. All the other doctors with whom I had spoken up until then agreed that the outlook for recovery of function of damaged brain cells was grim in the extreme.

As well, I had seen the devastating effects that a brain injured child could have on the family, resulting in well documented high rates of family breakdown, divorce, and an increased incidence of emotional and social disorder in the other siblings. In fact, the medical school that I attended had a special interest in this area. So drastic were the effects on the family that the department of child care encouraged parents to admit such children to hospital care on a semi-permanent basis. According to my lecture notes of that time (1976), this was done to 'give the parents a rest, to allow the family to develop normally, and to reduce the alarmingly high rate of social pathology in these sadly affected people'. Fortunately, attitudes to this well-meant process of 'institutionalizing' brain injured children are changing rapidly as the adverse social, economic and emotional effects of this policy become evident to the community.

I can well remember watching some brain injured children in the physiotherapy department of a teaching hospital. The consultant gently closed the door before saying: 'Of course, there is nothing that can be done for these poor children. As you are well aware, no nervous tissue regeneration can take place, but at least this way we are offering the parents some emotional support so that they can gradually get used to the idea that these patients are irretrievable'. Please remember that this was said in kindness and great sorrow by a world-famous paediatrician still in practice in a very well known hospital.

Statements such as these represent the limit of training that doctors receive in the long-term care of brain injured children. I was taught that the only hope was for children whose IQs were above 50 – they would receive special schooling because they could become reasonably independent as adults. However, I was taught about the medical aspects of the treatment of brain injury – the emergency care in the neo-natal and intensive care wards.

Unfortunately, there is a price to be paid for the type of didactic training that most medical students receive. There is a striking lack of independent thought among most doctors, together with a reluctance to use their critical faculties when confronted with new theories that have yet to be substantiated by the proper medical authorities. With a justifiable fear of doing harm, many doctors hide their heads in the sands of caution, and they are unwilling to test or examine evidence that may challenge existing theories.

So parents of brain injured children probably have to deal with doctors trained as I was. As well, if the doctor is working in a group practice, he has to justify his decisions to his partners – also didactically trained. Thus, it is little wonder that he does not feel too confident about recommending alternative treatments or therapies, especially since the word 'alternative' still carries overtones of 'quackery', 'deviant' and 'odd'.

On top of this, the doctor is trying to do his best for a patient whose parents have been through one of life's worst experiences. He would expect them to be highly emotionally charged, since they are faced with the bleak, although usually unspoken message: 'We can do no more'. They may also be going through what Elizabeth Kubler-Ross refers to in *On Death and Dying*[1] as the angry stage of grief. Sometimes these people are collapsing emotionally with all they have to deal with. The doctor can see no point in raising their hopes with something he knows little about and which runs contrary to his knowledge of brain injury. If the therapy was tried and was unsuccessful, he would then have to deal with the consequences of this failure – something which may be more than the already over-burdened parents can deal with. Upset and disappointed parents may cause scenes that the doctor would wish to avoid. As well, he may be blamed or even sued for the failure. It is often thought easier for everyone if the doctor retreats to safe ground – the non-challenging *status quo*.

This description of what is probably going through a doctor's mind when he considers the prospect of alternative therapy for a brain injured child will hopefully give you an insight into the typical GP's or paediatrician's decision-making processes and fears. An understanding of how the doctor may react is of great value if you are going to handle the situation properly.

In my case, the first contact with a brain injured patient caused me to remember something I had read in a book on positive thinking: 'Always challenge and think for yourself'. So, this appeared to be the time to put such advice into action. I began to look again at the whole issue of brain injury and recovery of function. I recalled seeing war veterans who had lost great portions of their brains, and yet had relearnt how to read and write. I had seen stroke victims gradually recover a great deal of their function. I now thought of these examples of seemingly miraculous recovery, and began to wonder how it had happened.

It seemed that these examples directly challenged my original teaching which had said that little or no progress could occur following brain injury. After reading scientific reports of partial regeneration of rat brains following deliberate injury and the migration of cells within injured rat brains, it seemed clear that compensatory and repair mechanisms were present in the rat brain. Therefore, at least from a theoretical point of view, I was prepared to accept that it was possible that similar mechanisms may be present in the human brain, and that these could be brought into action following brain injury – the stroke patients and war victims seemed to suggest this. Thus, I approached the question of alternative therapy with an open mind – 'prove it to me' became my attitude.

But then, the next problem I had to deal with was that of the parents' emotions. They had come to me because their own doctor and specialists had rejected out of hand their interest in alternative therapy. Despite the fact that the parents had seen a consultant paediatrician and a paediatric neurologist, their inquiries were dismissed in an unsympathetic and rather irrational manner. One of the specialists I spoke to had seen a journal article that was critical of this new type of therapy, and on this basis felt prepared to stand in judgement of this method and advise the parents strongly against it. Neither specialist had read in detail the literature objectively describing the therapy; they had not seen the therapy in action, had not seen first hand how it affected the rest of the family, nor had they directly contacted anyone involved in the organization that was administering the therapy.

In the cases where the doctors advise against the therapy program, the parents often do it in secret. Although the doctor may see improvement in the child, he is unaware that this is due to the therapy the child has been undergoing – therefore his attitude does not change. As strange as it may seem, some doctors in this situation appear uninterested in finding out why the child has made more progress than he would have expected. Many parents have recounted a situation where the doctor has been pleased, and sometimes amazed, with the child's improvement and yet there was no attempt made to discover the reason for what had happened to the child.

The parents who came to me were sensible and logical about their desire to try alternative therapy – their attitude was: 'There's nothing else to be done, so why not give it a go?' Also, they appeared to have a good marriage and a stable home environment. The thing that concerned me most was the effect the therapy program would have on the other children – with so many people coming into their house to help with the program and giving all their attention to the one child, I felt that it would be difficult for them to have a normal childhood. However, I have noticed that since the therapy was begun, the parents' morale has increased so much that they have been able to properly care for the other children. I have not seen any evidence of the siblings suffering emotional damage – in fact, to the contrary, the family has become closer and its members more caring of each other.

So, after much consideration, I said to the parents: 'Do it if you really want to. I would be interested in observing the program and monitoring the effects on the child and the family.' I did give one warning: 'Be prepared to stop if at any time I feel it is doing more harm than good.' I knew that the family would have done the therapy regardless, so I felt it was better to at least offer them support. I was impressed by their quiet determination to get the best for their child in the face of apparently hopeless odds. On reading the details of the therapy program the child was eventually given, I was further assured by the thought that the child would not be made any worse by the therapy. Indeed, it was a great deal less onerous than the training schedules for young ballet dancers, gymnasts or athletes.

Thus, both the parents and myself, as the child's doctor, were quite happy with the trust and working relationship we had established. How can other parents achieve a similar satisfactory arrangement? It is best to approach a general practitioner first as you may need to be referred to a specialist; also, since there are so many GPs, you are more likely to discover at least some independent thought. But this cannot be guaranteed, as you may come up against someone safely entrenched in didactic thought. If this happens, be prepared to keep looking for the right person, even if this means a lot of travelling for people living in the country.

The doctor's surgery may give you further clues. Look around – has there been an attempt to humanize the room? Has the doctor placed the patients' chairs directly in front of the desk in what can

be interpreted as a confrontationist attitude, or has he some awareness of the importance of body language and had the confidence to
place you diagonally, or even with no desk between you and him?
You will probably find dialogue with such a person much easier, and
while he may not accept your ideas, he is more likely to give you a
good hearing, or point you to a doctor who may receive you more
enthusiastically.

If you have not been to the doctor before, recite your child's
problems in a calm, unemotional way, for too much emotion may be
seen as a sign of irrational judgement. State that you have come to
him because you have been dissatisfied with the attitude of the
other doctors you have seen, but do not criticize these doctors as
they may be friends of his, and he must be professionally loyal. You
should then follow the procedure laid out in the previous chapter –
leave him information about the therapy program, and come back
for an extended appointment to discuss the whole issue.

This may sound puerile and even didactic, but if you want to be
taken seriously, you must adopt a business-like manner. If the doctor sees your rational determination, he is unlikely to simply pass
you off as an over-emotional parent grasping at straws. If you can
manage to have your spouse or partner present, so much the better, as it shows good teamwork and a solid relationship with mutual
commitment to a project.

A word of warning – make sure you keep copies of your information, in case the doctor throws the whole lot in the bin! Don't
give up though, for there are lots of splendid doctors who have open
minds, and they nearly all want to do what is best for you. But
remember that doctors are people first, and it is human nature for
some people to be naturally 'closed-minded'. Happily, there is a
wind of change blowing through medicine, and more and more doctors are beginning to assess different forms of therapy in a more
positive light. Keep trying and good luck!

Section VII
A Happy Ending

CHAPTER THIRTY-THREE

It Really Can Work!

IN THIS book, we have told the stories of five children – Chantal, Ryan, Terese, Duncan and Kevin. They were stories of heartbreak and despair, of gloomy prospects and little hope, typical of what most people would perceive to be the sad world of brain injured children.

However, we do not believe it always has to be this way, and we have seen results that prove this. As a way of demonstrating what can be done, let us look at what has happened to each of the five children. In normal circumstances, it would be expected that in the story of the lives of these brain injured children the next chapter would be as depressing as the first. However, as you will soon see, this is not the case. In fact, each child has made remarkable progress. Their futures now look much brighter than first predicted.

But how much progress was due to the treatment program they underwent? What would have happened to them if they had not done it? Obviously, these questions can never be answered, since who can tell how a child would have developed without therapy. And yet, on many occasions parents whose children have made good progress due to intensive therapy are told: 'It would have happened anyway'. Often the person saying this is the doctor who, two years earlier, told the parents not to expect significant progress. Of course, the parents walk out of the doctor's office flabbergasted and amazed at this sudden change in attitude. What frustrates them most is that they cannot prove their hard work was responsible for the child's progress.

It seems more than just coincidence that in most cases, the child progressed only after the treatment program had begun. In fact, the reason most parents decide to undertake an intensive program is because the child's progress, up until that time, has been too slow or non-existent. If the child improves far beyond the expectations of the professionals, expectations that are based on what has happened to similar children, it would seem reasonable to assume that the treatment program was at least partially responsible. Credit needs to be given where credit is due.

Although Chantal, Ryan, Terese, Duncan and Kevin have made remarkable progress, this does not mean that all children who undergo this type of treatment will do as well. Just because it works with one child does not mean it will work with another. However, what it does demonstrate is that there is hope, that there is a chance that progress can be made. After continually being told how poorly brain injured children develop, it is about time that parents were told that these children can improve, and improve well. Instead of dwelling on past failures, it should be realized that something *can* be done.

These stories are a suitable testimony to both the parents and children involved. They show what love, determination, and lots of hard work can achieve in the face of great adversity.

(Reference is made to ACBIC in these stories – this is the Australian Centre for Brain Injured Children, the organization that directed the treatment programs.)

Duncan

Remember Duncan? He was the autistic child, whose mother, Jenny, had desperately tried to find someone to recognize that her son had a problem, and that something needed to be done about it. Jenny has written his story in two parts – the first being what she imagines it would have been like if she had taken everyone's advice and just accepted Duncan the way he was. The second describes what happened because of her refusal to accept this.

Duncan's future without an ACBIC start

When Duncan was aged two years, the medical people I was seeing suggested that I should prepare myself for the future. I should start thinking of placing him in an institution, where there were people who were trained to handle children with special needs. I was told that these people could take proper care of him, thus taking the burden away from me.

Duncan *was* aggressive, the doctors were right. He was also a strong two-year-old. He had proved his strength by throwing wooden blocks through window panes on many occasions. He even jerked his head forward once while I was cuddling him, and I ended up with a broken nose. I was told that he was deaf, and that he probably would not be toilet trained for years. He did not walk, and could not even crawl on his hands and knees. It was painfully clear to me that his one joy was to sleep, and when he was awake he would merely stare at a burning light globe, and would yell if interrupted from his hypnotic gaze.

My life was *so* miserable and my family suffered terribly. We were all very unhappy. You would think in this situation, it would be a simple solution to place Duncan in an institution. We would always love him, even if he didn't know it. Life goes on – doesn't it?

Nobody knows how a mother hurts for her handicapped child – that is, nobody but another mother in the same predicament. I don't blame anyone who decides to place their severely handicapped or retarded child in the hands of professionals. But, I know that if I had taken that step with Duncan, he would have just slept happily along, being well cared for, and he would never be hungry or cold. He would have definitely needed large doses of tranquillizers to control his outrageous tantrums. Duncan my little pumpkin – just a pumpkin. He would have lived up to all the doctors' predictions – autistic, deaf and uncontrollable.

Duncan's life with an ACBIC start

Duncan is now nine-years-old, and he attends the Bulleen Special School, a school for mildly handicapped children. He is learning, and he can be educated. He can count to 50, recite the alphabet, and his drawings are meaningful and really quite good. He can even play football, although his knowledge of the rules is limited. He is an important member of his school, and he loves to feel involved with any special tasks.

At home, Duncan is my little soldier. He loves television, especially the Muppets, and I just adore to hear him laughing. His latest conquest is swimming under water – what a guy!

My little man is bursting with health and happiness, and is really switched on to life. He has many friends, both adult and children, and I really think that they have benefited from knowing him. They enjoy helping him to reach his goals, with every achievement being a giant step.

Nobody knows what Duncan's future will be. But, I ask you, who knows what is ahead for any child? I do know one thing – he is not in an institution, and he does not need to take medication. He has leapt over many barriers, and he now has a chance to lead a good life.

My Duncan is a 'normal' child who has a few problems, but he is working on these. His main difficulty is speech and understanding, although I believe that one day he will be able to talk normally. All right, he is 'handicapped', but only mildly so, and he is improving all the time. As well, he is home with his family, and we just love him so.

ACBIC was my last resort, for there was simply nothing else available. When you compare my description of what would have happened to Duncan without the program, and what he is like today, all the hard work involved during two and a half years of therapy seems like nothing.

ACBIC showed me how to reach my son when all else failed.

Chantal

Chantal, if you remember, was diagnosed as being blind, and her overall development was expected to be extremely limited. However, Kerrie, her mother, tells a very different story to what we would expect:

Next week, Chantal starts her schooling at the Orana Special School for handicapped children. She is now five years old, and is so different to the child the doctors told us to expect. As amazing as it may seem, she now has *normal* vision. Not only can she see very well, but she is even able to read 50 words!

When we first started the program, she couldn't even roll over – now she can walk, and is starting to run. She was unaware of her body, but now she shows great interest in all its different parts. The most exciting recent development is that she is beginning to communicate her wishes and feelings, and she has many recognizable words of speech. Her present level of understanding is probably equal to that of a two-and-a-half-year-old. What a contrast this is to the predictions that her understanding would never develop beyond the level of a one-year-old.

It has been a long road to get this far, and it hasn't been easy. But the results make it all worthwhile. We were far better off having a positive, intensive program to concentrate on, rather than the small amount of physiotherapy that was suggested to us in the beginning. Although it offered no promises, at least the ACBIC program gave us something hopeful to work with. It was so much better to at least have hope, for it gave us the energy and motivation to do what needed to be done.

All the negative thoughts are now gone, the nightmare has disappeared. Instead, we look forward to the future with hope and enjoyment, in the knowledge that Chantal should continue to progress and develop. ACBIC offered a glimmer of hope in an otherwise dark and never-ending tunnel.

Ryan

Ryan's biggest problem was different to those of the other children whom we have discussed, for it was not directly related to his brain injury. As a result of a structural problem, his spine was severely twisted and malformed, a condition known as scoliosis. It was so severe that he was not expected to live very long. In addition, he suffered developmental problems related to his brain injury. As his mother Jan tells us, not only did he survive, but he has continued to progress way beyond everybody's expectations:

We recently saw our paediatrician for a six-monthly check-up, and he continues to be amazed at Ryan's progress. From a medical viewpoint, the improvement has been quite incredible. One of our main reasons for initially starting the therapy program was the very real fear that Ryan would die from pneumonia. He had had many upper respiratory infections and one severe attack of pneumonia up until that time, and the doctors had warned us that this would be a continuing problem. And yet, in the two and a half years since we began the therapy, Ryan has had absolutely no major respiratory problems. The paediatrician was so pleased that he told us we could now start looking at long-term goals for Ryan – he had not talked about the future before, simply because he didn't expect Ryan to survive. My local doctor told me later that a letter he had received from the paediatrician had praised our work, devotion and perseverance with Ryan, and said that this was directly responsible for his amazing progress.

Naturally we were elated to hear this, and so have continued working hard with Ryan. He improved so much that last year we were able to place him in a normal kindergarten, something we had thought unlikely when we were first told of his problems. He did so well that we were advised to set our sights on sending him to school. We wanted him to go to a normal school, but we came up against unexpected opposition. The local school refused to take him, even though they accepted that he was very intelligent. The nearest crippled children's school was an hour-and-a-quarter's drive away, and the orthopaedic surgeon advised us that travelling so far would worsen his spine.

However, all our plans seemed shattered after one of Ryan's regular visits to the orthopaedic specialist. Until that time, he had been pleased with Ryan's progress, but now he informed us that the spine had worsened. It was becoming rigid and was now in a dangerous position. This meant that an operation would most likely be needed, otherwise he could become a quadriplegic, and then possibly die from lung failure due to pressure from his spine.

We were stunned. Although we had always known that Ryan would probably need surgery, we were terrified of this prospect. For, unless he was strong enough, the doctors had informed us that his chances of surviving the extensive surgery were not good. They had wanted to delay the operation for as long as possible, in the hope that his condition would improve. But now it seemed they had no choice.

Although recognizing the need for surgery, the orthopaedic surgeon was very pleased with the condition that Ryan was in. He said that two years ago, he could not have even considered surgery. Even if it was necessary, at that time Ryan was so weak and floppy, and full of mucus, that he would not have survived the operation. But, as a result of all our hard work, he felt that Ryan had improved 300 per cent since he first saw him. As he was continuing to improve, the surgeon felt that it would be possible to delay the surgery a little further.

Meanwhile, we had to speak to the paediatrician and the anaesthetist to get their permission for the operation, as Ryan's respiratory system was not normal. We were told that there was a 20 per cent risk that he might not survive the surgery, since he might not be able to breathe by himself afterwards, or he might contract an infection; however both specialists advised us to go ahead with the surgery whenever it was necessary, as long as we realized that there were risks involved. We were pleased that these doctors were able to recommend the surgery, since it was because they had seen tremendous progress in our little boy. We saw the orthopaedic surgeon three months later, and this time his news was more encouraging. Again, due to all the hard work we were doing, he felt that the spine still had some elasticity, and therefore it would not be necessary to do the surgery in the immediate future. Hopefully, if Ryan continues to progress as he has, the surgery can be delayed for even longer.

Although we were hoping to delay his operation until he was much older, we feel that at least we have given him a chance to live – a chance that his doctors had previously thought unlikely. He can at least undergo the surgery with a 70 to 80 per cent possibility of surviving. Before we did the therapy program, he had a 70 to 80 per cent chance of dying. We feel that we have achieved our goal, and will continue working with him until the surgery forces us to stop. He has overcome so many obstacles so far, we are making sure we are doing all we can to ensure that he will make it through this, his biggest one. An added bonus for us is the recent news that another local normal school has accepted Ryan on a part-time basis.

Terese

After being told that not much could be expected of their daughter Terese, her parents, Kris and Rob have achieved much more than even they thought was possible:

After first visiting ACBIC, our attitudes towards our daughter and her future changed drastically. No longer were we always dwelling on the desperate picture that had been described to us by all the doctors we had visited. Now, at least, some hope was given that she may improve. For the first time we were able to look into the future without being overwhelmed by fear and despair. In fact, we were excited with the prospect of getting the therapy program under way.

Since Terese was only three and a half months old at the time we first started, we had some difficulty with the people who offered to help us, as they were naturally wary of working with such a young baby. But once we explained that her young age was in fact an advantage, they soon overcame their initial fears and the program began in earnest.

We were advised to recruit people to assist us with the treatment, both to share the workload and provide Terese with added stimulation. We were a little reluctant to do this in the beginning, as we are both quite independent and, as we had just moved into the neighbourhood, we didn't know many people. To begin with, Terese's uncle and great aunt called on all the houses in a one block radius, requesting assistance to help with the program. The response was amazing, for even before they returned home, the phone began ringing, and offers of assistance from people we had never met came flooding in. This support was very important in helping us cope with the problems at hand, and it made us feel that we were not alone. As well, it taught us an important lesson about the basic goodness of human nature.

As the months went by, our hopes were beginning to come true, for Terese was responding to the treatment. It was so terribly exciting for us to see her developing and achieving the goals that were set for her. It seemed almost too good to be true. However, it was not all plain sailing. At times, Terese would play up, and it would be difficult to work with her. At other times it would seem that we were getting nowhere, and all the hard work would become a drudgery. But then Terese would achieve something new, and the excitement of watching her use this new function made everything worthwhile.

So significant was her progress that at the end of eighteen months, we felt that she was developing well enough to no longer need the constant stimulation. Therefore, we decided to take her off the program to see how she would go. We still kept up different kinds of intellectual input, but she was basically left to her own devices. Much to our delight, she continued to progress, and has never looked back. This year she started at the local public school for normal children!

We do not know how she will cope in this school, as she still has speech problems, but we are simply amazed that she was able to go there in the first place. In those horrible days after we learnt of her problem, we never imagined, even in our wildest dreams, that we would ever feel as proud of her as we do today.

Terese is a very determined little girl, very loving and full of life. She has developed her own personality and has taken her place in a world that we were told she didn't belong in. We will never be able to say what it was that got her so far, for human development is not yet a science where absolutes can be determined, predicted and measured. What we do know is that, given the gift of hindsight, we would not change a thing we did in the last five years since Terese's birth. Our whole family is richer and more united for the experience.

KEVIN

Remember Kevin? No one really thought he would get any better after he came out of coma following his near-drowning. But his mother, Gemma, thought otherwise and was determined to do all she could to try and get her son back again.

Some time after Kevin's accident, it was suggested we undertake physiotherapy with him in an effort to combat the rigidity of his limbs. The hospital was almost an hour's drive away, but for eighteen months I struggled to take Kevin for daily treatment.

The one-hour sessions were conducted haphazardly and were often interrupted, so you never got the full time allocated, which wasn't much anyway. There didn't seem to be a set program you could follow up at home, and it was never suggested that this would be a good idea. Anyway, by the time I had negotiated the city traffic with a severely handicapped child, and coped with parking, wheelchairs, hospital waiting rooms, over-worked therapists, and the long, often bitterly sad drive home, I wasn't in any frame of mind to pursue further therapy, even if I had known what to do. And I couldn't neglect the rest of the family whom I also loved and who needed me. There just weren't enough hours in the day.

After Kevin's accident, my sister suggested I get in touch with ACBIC as she had heard of their work. I discussed this with Kevin's therapist and he strongly advised me against trying the program. In fact, he scared the wits out of me, saying the hospital would accept no responsibility if anything happened to Kevin, and that he would probably get worse, not better. So I didn't pursue it.

I will be eternally sorry that I was so easily put off, because it took two and a half long, desperate years for me to finally get in touch with ACBIC. Time wasted while my beloved son made no progress other than losing his rigidity – only to turn into a floppy rag doll.

ACBIC was the first organization that gave me hope that there was a chance that Kevin could lead some sort of normal life. This was the first group that had a positive attitude. And it lifted my spirits enormously. I wasn't looking for a miracle cure, but just the thought that Kevin might get a little better was a miracle in itself.

Today, six years after starting the program, often doing up to eight hours of intensive therapy each day, the improvement in Kevin is vast. You simply would not believe he is the same boy who lay wrapped up in a bean bag, immobile and silent.

Now he can walk by himself – slowly and unsteadily – but walk non-etheless. Most of his current therapy is three to four hours daily of working on improving his walking. He can feed himself and go to the toilet alone. His level of understanding is right up to normal and he is completely aware of everything that is going on around him. He sees and hears well, but still has some trouble speaking clearly – although this continues to improve.

In terms of mental development – well, you've only got to look at his progress at school. He goes to the Catholic school down the road and loves it. He is doing extremely well with his work, and his teacher is very pleased with him. The children in his class are his own age, and he is able to keep up with them. He has lots of friends there and I think he is one of the best known kids in the school.

Last year, Friends (an ACBIC support network) bought him a home computer. And would you believe that this year, his thirty classmates have raised $300 – by selling five cent raffle tickets – to buy him a similar model to use in the classroom. That's a lot of raffle tickets, and evidence of how much everyone loves him.

Things do take him longer to do, naturally. It *is* harder for him to keep up. But we're all so proud of him. And so very happy with his progress. Kevin now has the prospect of a happy, fulfilling life ahead of him. And an independent life – that's important too. He has not only got a future, but a bright future.

The difficult I'll do right now,
The impossible will take a little while.

From the song 'Crazy He Calls Me'
By Carl Sigman and Sidney Keith Russell
(Harry Fox/Memory Lane)

References

Introduction

1 Figures from the Spastics Society
2 Figures from Mencap
3 Figures from the National Society for Autistic Children
4 These figures do not include those suffering from mental illness
5 United Cerebral Palsy Association, USA, personal correspondence
6 Australian Brain Foundation brochure, *Head injury: a layman's guide*
7 National Head Injury Foundation (USA) brochure, *Help for the head injured and their families*
8 Dan N. G., 'The epidemiology of neurotrauma', in *Modern Medicine Australia*, 26:6, 1983

Chapter 3

1 Guilfoyle, E. A., Grady, A. P. and Moore, J. C., *Children Adapt*, Charles Slack, New Jersey, 1981

Chapter 4

1 Black, P. (Ed), *Brain Dysfunction in Children*, New York, Raven Press, 1981
2 Ulleland, C. N., Wennberg, R. P., Igo, R. P. and Smith, N. J., 'The offspring of alcoholic mothers', in *Paediatric Research*, 1970, 4:474

Chapter 5

1 Nauta, W.J.H. and Feirtag, M., 'The organization of the brain', in *Scientific American*, 241:3, 1979
2 Barr, M. L., *The Human Nervous System*, 2nd ed., New York, Harper & Row, 1974
3 Granit, R., *The Purposive Brain*, Cambridge, MIT Press, 1977
4 Buzan, T., *Use Both Sides of Your Brain*, New York, E. P. Dutton, 1976
5 Jacobson, M., *Developmental Neurobiology*, 2nd ed., New York, Plenum Press, 1978
6 Hirsch, H.V.B. and Jacobson, M., 'The perfectible brain – principles of

neuronal development', in *Handbook of Psychobiology*, Gazzaniga, M. S., Blakemore, C. (Eds), New York, Academic Press, 1975

7 Luria, A. R., Naydin, V. L., Tsvetkova, L. S. and Vinarskaya, E. N., 'Restoration of higher cortical function following local brain damage', in *Handbook of Clinical Neurology*, Vol 3, Vinken, P. J., Bruyer, G. W. (Eds), Amsterdam, North Holland Publishing Company, 1969

Chapter 6

1 Granit, R., *The Purposive Brain*, Cambridge, MIT Press, 1977

2 Brodal, A., 'The wiring patterns of the brain' in *The Neurosciences: Paths of Discovery*, Worden, F. P., Swazey, J. P., Adelman, G. (Eds), Cambridge, MIT Press, 1975

3 Bach-y-Rita, P., 'Brain plasticity as a basis for therapeutic procedures' in *Recovery of Function: Theoretical Considerations for Brain Injury Rehabilitation*, Bach-y-Rita, P. (Ed), Bern, Huber, 1980

4 Flohr, H. and Precht, W. (Eds), *Lesion-induced Neuronal Plasticity in Sensorimotor Systems*, Berlin, Springer-Verlag, 1981

5 Lorber, Le Winn, R., as discussed in 'Is your brain really necessary?', in *Science*, 210:1232-1234, 1980

6 Glees, P., 'Functional reorganization following hemispherectomy in man and after small experimental lesions in primates', in *Recovery of Function: Theoretical Considerations for Brain Injury Rehabilitation*, Bach-y-Rita, P. (Ed), Bern, Huber, 1980

7 Luria, A. R., *Restoration of Function After Brain Injury*, New York, Macmillan, 1963

8 Sameroff, A. J. and Chandler, M. J., 'Reproductive risk and the continuum of caretaker casualty', in Horowitz, F. D. (Ed), *Review of Child Development*, Vol 4, Chicago, University of Chicago Press, 1975

9 Stein, D. G. and Lewis, M. E., 'Functional recovery after brain damage in adult organisms', in Vital-Durand, F. and Jeannerod, M. (Eds), *Aspects of neural plasticity*, Paris, Editions INSERM, Vol 43, 1975

10 Stein, D. G. and Schultze, M., 'Recovery of function in the albino rat following either simultaneous or serial lesions of the candate nucleus', in *Experimental Neurology*, 46:291-301, 1975

11 Ayers, A. J., *Sensory Integration and Learning Disorders*, Los Angeles, Western Psychological Services, 1972

12 Moore, J., 'Neuroanatomical considerations relating to recovery of function following brain injury', in Bach-y-Rita, P. (Ed), *Recovery of Function: Theoretical Considerations for Brain Injury Rehabilitation*, Bern, Huber, 1980

13 Lui, C. N. and Chambers, W. W., 'Intraspinal sprouting of dorsal route axons', in *Archives of Neurology*, 79:46-61, 1958

14 Guth, L., 'Axonal regeneration and functional plasticity in the central nervous system', in *Experimental Neurology*, 45:606-654, 1969

15 Devor, M., 'Neuroplasticity in the sparing or deterioration of function after early olfactory tract lesions', in *Science*, 190:998-1000, 1975

16 Cottman, C. W. and Scheff, S. W., 'Compensatory synapse growth in aged animals after neuronal death', in Mech.Age.Dev., 9:103-117, 1979

17 Matthews, D. E., Cottman, C. W. and Lynch, G., 'An electron microscopic study of lesion-induced synaptogenesis in the denate gyrus of the adult rat: reappearance of morphologically normal synaptic contacts,' in *Brain Research*, 115:23-41, 1976

18 Schneider, G. E., 'Early lesions of superior colliculus: factors affecting the formation of abnormal retinal projections', in *Brain Behaviour in Evolution*, 8:73-109, 1973

19 Kerr, F.L.W., 'Structural and functional evidence of plasticity in the central nervous system', in *Experimental Neurology*, 48:16-31, 1975

20 Isaacson, R. L., 'Recovery (?) from early brain damage', in *Aberrant Development in Infancy*, Ellis, N. E. (Ed), London, Wiley, 1976

21 Lynch, G., Deadwyler, S. and Cottman, C. W., 'Postlesion axonal growth produces permanent functional connections', in *Science*, 180:1364-1366, 1973

22 Wall, P. D., 'Mechanisms of plasticity of connection following damage in adult mammalian nervous systems', in *Recovery of Function: Theoretical Considerations for Brain Injury Rehabilitation*, Bach-y-Rita, P. (Ed), Bern, Huber, 1980

23 Saint James-Roberts, I., 'Neurological plasticity, recovery from brain insult, and child development', in *Advances in Child Development and Behaviour*, 14:253-319, 1979

24 Rosenzweig, M. R., 'Effects of environment on development of brain and behaviour', in *The Biopsychology of Development*, Tobach, E., Aronson, L., Shaw, E. (Eds), New York, Academic Press, 1971

25 Goldman, P. S. and Lewis, M. E., 'Developmental biology of brain damage and experience', in *Neuronal Plasticity*, Cottman, C. W. (Ed), New York, Raven Press, 1978

26 Rosenzweig, M. R., 'Animal models for effects of brain lesions and for rehabilitation', in *Recovery of Function:Theoretical Considerations for Brain Injury Rehabilitation*, Bach-y-Rita, P. (Ed), Bern, Huber, 1980

27 Bennett, E. L., Diamond, M. C., Kresch, D. and Rosenzweig, M. R., 'Chemical and anatomical plasticity of brain', in *Science*, 146:610-619, 1964

28 Rosenzweig, M. R., Bennett, E. L. and Diamond, M. C., 'Brain changes in response to experience', in *Scientific American*, 226(2):22-29, 1972

29 Rosenzweig, M. R., and Bennett, E. L., 'Experiential influences on brain anatomy and brain chemistry in rodents', in *Studies on the Development of Behaviour and the Nervous System, Vol 4, Early Influences*, Gottlieb, G. (Ed), Academic Press, New York, 1978

30 Blakemore, C., 'Development of functional connections in the mammalian visual system', in *British Medical Bulletin*, 30:152-157, 1974

31 Grobstein, P. and Chow, K. L., 'Receptive field development and individual experience', in *Science*, 190:352-358, 1975

32 Hubel, D. H., Wiesel, T. N. and Le Vay, S., 'Plasticity of ocular dominance columns in monkey striate cortex', in *Phil.Trans., Royal Society of London Bulletin*, 278:377-410, 1977

33 Schwartz, S., 'Effects of neonatal cortical lesions and early environmental factors on adult rat behaviour', in *Journal of Comparative Physiology and Psychology*, 57:72-77, 1964
34 Will, B. E., Rosenzweig, M.R. and Bennett, E.L., 'Effects of differential environments on recovery from neonatal brain lesions, measured by problem-solving scores and brain dimensions', in *Physiology of Behaviour*, 16:603-611, 1975
35 Will, B. E., Rosenzweig, M. R., Bennett, E. L. Herbert, M. and Morimoto, H., 'Relatively brief environmental enrichment aids recovery of learning capacity and alters brain measures after postweaning brain lesions', in *Journal of Comparative Physiology and Psychology*, 91:33-50, 1977
36 Will, B. E., 'Methods for promoting functional recovery following brain damage', in *Brain, Fetal and Infant: Current Research on Normal and Abnormal Development*, Berenberg, S. R. (Ed), Amsterdam, Martinus Nijhoff, 1978
37 White, B. L. and Held, R., 'Plasticity and sensorimotor development in the human infant', in *The Causes of Behaviour: Readings in Child Development and Education Psychology*, Rosenblith, J. F. & Allinsmith, W. (Eds), Boston, Allyn and Bacon, 1966
38 White, B. L., 'An experimental approach to the effects of experience on early human behaviour', in *Minnesota Symposium on Child Psychology*, Minneapolis, University of Minnesota Press, 1967

Chapter 8

1 Teitelbaum, P., Cheng, M. and Rozin, P., 'Development of feeding parallels its recovery after hypothalamic damage', in *Journal of Comparative Physiology and Psychology*, 67:4, 430-441, 1969
2 Teitelbaum, P., Cheng, M. and Rozin, P., 'Stages of recovery and development of lateral hypothalamic control of food and water intake', in *Annals of the New York Academy of Science*, 157:2, 849-858, 1967
3 Twitchell, T. E., 'The automatic grasping responses of infants', in *Neuropsychologia*, 3, 247-259, 1965
4 Twitchell, T. E., 'Reflex mechanisms and the development of prehension', in Connolly, K. J., (Ed), *Mechanisms of Motor Skill Development*, New York, Academic Press, 25-38, 1970
5 Teitelbaum, P., 'The use of recovery of function to analyze the organization of motivated behaviour in the nervous system', in *Neurosciences Research Program Bulletin*, 12:2, 255-260, 1974
6 Ommaya, A. K., 'Trauma to the nervous system', in *Annals of the Royal College of Surgeons*, England, 39:317-347, 1966
7 Raisman, G., 'What hope for repair of the brain?', in *Annals of Neurology*, 3:101-106, 1978
8 Moore, J., 'Neuroanatomical considerations relating to recovery of function following brain injury', in Bach-y-Rita, P. (Ed): *Recovery of Function:*

Theoretical Considerations for Brain Injury Rehabilitation, Bern, Huber, 1980

Chapter 9

1 Rose, S., *The Conscious Brain*, Middlesex, Pelican Books, 1976
2 Smith, D. W., *Recognizable Patterns of Human Malformation*, Philadelphia, W. B. Saunders Co., 1982
3 Kagan, J., 'Do infants think?', in *Scientific American*, 226:3, 1972
4 Piaget, J., *The Child's Construction of Reality*, New York, Routledge & Kegan Paul, 1955
5 Flavell, J. H., *The Developmental Psychology of Jean Piaget*, New York, Van Nostrand, 1963
6 Leach, P. J., *Babyhood*, 2nd Edition, Middlesex, Pelican Books, 1983
7 Caplan, F., *The First Twelve Months of Life*, New York, Bantam Books, 1973
8 *Australian Parents and Children Magazine*, Issue 11, June/July 1983, Sydney, Depin Pty Ltd
9 Montessori, M., *The Absorbent Mind*, New York, Dell Publishing Co., 1967

Chapter 10

1 Piaget, J., *The Origins of Intelligence in the Child*, New York, Routledge & Kegan Paul, 1953
2 Caplan, F., *The First Twelve Months of Life*, New York, Bantam Books, 1973
3 Fantz, R. L., 'Pattern discrimination and selective attention as determinants of perceptual development from birth', in Aline, J., Kidd, J., Rivoire, J. L. *Perceptual Development in Children*, London, University of London Press, 1966
4 Leach, P. J. *Baby and Child*, Middlesex, Penguin Books, 1977
5 Leach, P. J. *Babyhood*, Middlesex, Pelican Books, 1983
6 Atkinson, J., 'New tool pinpoints focusing fault in babies', in *New Scientist*, April 24, p.194, 1980

Chapter 11

1 Gesell, A., Ilg, F.L. and Ames, L. B., *Infant and Child in the Culture Today*, Revised edition, London, Hamish Hamilton, 1975
2 Koch, J., *Superbaby*, London, Orbis, 1982
3 Bower, T.G.R., 'Repetitive processes in child development', in *Scientific American*, 235(5):38-47, November 1976
4 Bower, T.G.R., *Human Development*, San Francisco, W. H. Freeman, 1978

5 Bower, T.G.R., *Development in Infancy*, San Francisco, W. H. Freeman, 1982
6 Butterworth, G. E., A review of 'A primer of infant development', in *Perception*, 7:363-364, 1978
7 Trevarthen, C., 'Growth of visuomotor coordination in infants', in *Journal of Human Movement Studies*, 1:57, 1975
8 Dodwell, P. C., Muir, D. and Di Franco, D., 'Responses of infants to visually presented objects', in *Science*, 194:209-211, 1976
9 Di Franco, D., Muir, D. W. and Dodwell, P. C., 'Reaching in very young infants', in *Perception*, 7:385-392, 1978
10 Bower, T.G.R., Dunkeld, J. and Wishart, J. G., 'Infant perception of visually presented objects', in *Science*, 203:1137-1138, 1979
11 Dodwell, P. C., Muir, D. W. and Di Franco, D., 'Reply to Bower et al.', in *Science*, 203:1138-1139, 1979
12 Leach, P., *Babyhood*, 2nd edition, Middlesex, Penguin, 1983

Chapter 12

1 Moore, J., 'Neuroanatomical considerations relating to recovery of function following brain injury', in Bach-y-Rita, P. (Ed), *Recovery of Function: Theoretical Considerations for Brain Injury Rehabilitation*, Bern, Huber, 1980
2 Ayers, A. J., *Sensory Integration and Learning Disorders*, Los Angeles, Western Psychological Services, 1975
3 Leach, P., *Babyhood*, 2nd edition, Middlesex, Pelican, 1983

Chapter 15

1 Zubeck, J. P. and Wilgosh, L., 'Prolonged immobilization of the body: Changes in performance and in the electroencephalogram', in *Science*, 142:306-308, 1963
2 Zubeck, J. P., Welch, G. and Saunders, M. G., 'Electroencephalographic changes during and after 14 days of perceptual deprivation', in *Science*, 139:490-492, 1963
3 Heron, W., in Solomon, P. (Ed), *Sensory Deprivation*. Cambridge, Harvard University Press, p.6, 1961
4 Hull, J. and Zubeck, J. P., in *Perceptual and Motor Skills*, 14, p.231, 1962
5 Vernon, J. et al., *Progress Report on Studies of Sensory Deprivation*, Published by U.S. Army Leadership Human Research Unit, Monterey, Calif., 1961

Chapter 16

1 Crossman, E.R.F.W., 'Theory of acquisition of speed-skill', in *Ergonomics*, 2:153-166, 1959

2 Kottke, F. J., 'From reflex to skill: The training of coordination', in *Archives of Physical Medicine and Rehabilitation*, 61:551-561, 1980

Chapter 17

1 *Guinness Book of Records*, Middlesex, Guinness Books, 1985
2 Jouvet, M., 'Coma and other disorders of consciousness' in Vinken & Bruyn (Ed), *Handbook of Clinical Neurology*. Amsterdam, North Holland Publishing Company, Vol 3, 62-79, 1969
3 Sprague, J. M., Levitt, M., Robson, K., Liu, C. N., Stellar, E. and Chambers, W. W., 'A neuroanatomical and behavioural analysis of the syndromes resulting from midbrain lemniscal and reticular lesions in the cat', in *Archives of Ital. Biology*, 101:225-295, 1963
4 French, J. D., and Magoun, H. W., 'Effects of chronic lesions in central cephalic brain-stems of monkeys', in *Archives of Neurology and Psychiatry*, 68:577-812, 1952
5 Lindsley, D. B., Schreiner, H. L., Knowles, B. D. and Magoun, H. W., 'Behavioural and EEG changes following chronic brain-stem lesions in the cat', in *Electroencephalograph Clinical Neurophysiology*, 2:483-495, 1950
6 Teasdale, G. and Jennett, B., 'Assessment of coma and impaired consciousness', in *Lancet*, 2:81-84, 1974
7 Overgaard, J., Hvid-Hansen, O. and Land, A. M., 'Prognosis after head injuries based on early clinical examination', in *Lancet*, 2:631-635, 1973
8 Collins English Dictionary, Sydney, William Collins, 1979
9 Le Winn, E. B., *The child in coma: Human Neurological Development: Past, Present and Future*, NASA Conference Publication 2603, pp 17-20, 1978
10 Ommaya, A. K., 'Trauma to the nervous system', in *Annals of the Royal College of Surgeons*, England, 39:317-347, 1966
11 Jennett B. et al., 'Severe head injury in three countries', in *Journal of Neurology, Neurosurgery and Psychiatry*, 40:291-298, 1977
12 Stover, S. L. and Zeiger, H. E., 'Head injury in children and teenagers: functional recovery correlated with the duration of coma', in *Archives of Physical Medicine and Rehabilitation*, 57, 5:201-205, 1976
13 Galbraith, S., Jennett, B. and Raisman, G., 'Recovery from coma and reinnervation rate', in *Lancet*, p.710, 1978
14 Eccles, J. C., 'The effects of use and disuse on synaptic function', in Delafresnaye, J. F. (Ed), *Brain Mechanisms and Learning*, Oxford, Blackwell Scientific Publications, 1961
15 Zubeck, J. P. and Wilgosh, L., 'Prolonged immobilization of the body: Changes in performance and in the electroencephalogram', in *Science*, 140:306-308, 1963

Chapter 21

1 Young, R. D., 'Effect of prenatal drugs and neonatal stimulation on later

behaviour', in *Journal of Comparative Physiology and Psychology*, 58:309-311, 1964

2 Levine, S., 'Some effects of stimulation in infancy', in Barnett, S. A. (ed.) *Lessons of animal behaviour for the clinician*, Little Club, in *Clinical Developmental Medicine* 7, 1962

3 Ayers, A. J., *Sensory Integration and Learning Disorders*, Los Angeles, Western Psychological Services, 1975

Chapter 25

1 Johnson, G. H., Pervis, G. A., Wallace, G. 'What nutrients do our infants really get?' in *Nutrition Today Society Journal*, Annapolis, 1982

2 Feingold, B. F., *Why your child is hyperactive*, New York, Random House, 1974

3 Commonwealth Department of Health (Australia) brochure, *Identifying Food Additives*, Australian Government Publishing Service, Canberra, 1985

4 Harrell, R. F., Capp, D. R., Ravitz, L. R., 'Can nutritional supplements help mentally retarded children? An exploratory study', in *Proceedings of the National Academy of Sciences*, 78:574-578, January 1981

5 Hartmann, P., 'Breastfeeding – the science of the art', in *Nursing Mothers Association of Australia Newsletter*, October/November, 1983, p. 3-9

6 Kamath, K. R., 'Advantages of breast feeding', in *Paediatric Clinics of North America*, April, 1985, 32:2.

7 Anderson, G. H., 'Human milk feeding', in *Paediatric Clinics of North America*, April 1985, 32:2

8 Reynolds, G. J., 'Milk for premature babies', in *Nursing Mothers Association of Australia Newsletter*, January/February, 1984, p. 3-7

Chapter 27

1 Brain, Lord, *Brain's Clinical Neurology*, revised by Bannister, R., Oxford, Oxford University Press, 1978

2 Debakan, A. S., *Neurology of early childhood*. Baltimore, Williams & Wilkins, 1970

3 Debakan, A. S., 'Idiopathic epilepsy in early infancy: the question of frequent daily attacks causing undifferentiated type of mental deficiency', in *American Journal of Disabled Children*, 100:181-188, 1960

4 Alvarez W. C., *Nerves in Collision*, New York, Pyramid, 1972

Chapter 29

1 Wright, S., personal correspondence

Chapter 32

1 Kubler-Ross, E., *On Death and Dying*, Tavistock Publishing, New York, 1969

APPENDIX ONE

Australian Centre for Brain Injured Children (ACBIC) Questionnaire

Questionnaire sent in November 1983 to parents whose children were brain injured and who had received treatment from ACBIC for at least one year:

Total number sent 263
Number of completed questionnaires received 154
Number moved address and not contactable 27
Percentage return rate 65%

Relevant questions and answers (total of 28 questions asked)
Question 1: What age was your child when a problem was first suspected?
Answer: For the purposes of this questionnaire, this question was relevant only to those children brain injured from birth. Therefore, of the 154 respondents, those brain injured from any kind of trauma or illness after birth, or from a genetic disorder were eliminated (38 traumatic, 18 genetic), leaving a total of 100 children. Of these 100, 45 were detected within the first six months, 36 from six to 12 months, and 19 after 12 months.
Question 2: Who was the first person to raise the suspicion that something was wrong?
Answer: Of the 100 children brain injured from birth, 69 had their problems first detected by their parents, 6 by other family members, and 25 by a professional person. In the 69 cases where the problems were first noticed by the parents, 42% were detected in the first 6 months of the child's life, 36% from 6-12 months, and 22% after 12 months.
Question 23: How beneficial was the ACBIC treatment program for your child? The parents were asked to tick one of the following

categories: Very beneficial; Moderately beneficial; A little beneficial; Not at all beneficial; May have been harmful.

Answer:		
Very beneficial	83	53.9%
Moderately beneficial	43	27.9%
A little beneficial	24	15.6%
Not at all beneficial	2	1.3%
May have been harmful	2	1.3%

Question 27: How did the intensity of the ACBIC program affect your family? The parents were asked to tick one of the following choices: Positive effect on family unit; No effect, either adverse or positive; There were mild family problems; There were major family problems.

Answer: 146 parents responded to this question:

Positive effect on family unit	57	39%
No effect, positive or negative	16	11%
Mild family problems	61	42%
Major family problems	12	8%

APPENDIX TWO

The following centre carries out treatment based on the principles described in this book:

AUSTRALIA
Australian Centre for Brain Injured Children (ACBIC)
52-54 Argyle Street,
St. Kilda 3182
Telephone: (03) 534 8734

The following centres carry out treatment based on the principles described in this book, although they are not associated with the author or with the Australian Centre for Brain Injured Children:

GREAT BRITAIN
The British Institute for Brain-Injured Children,
Knowle Hall,
Knowle,
Bridgwater,
Somerset TA7 8PJ
Telephone: (0278) 684060

The Kerland Child Development Centre,
Marsh Lane,
Huntworth Gate,
Bridgwater,
Somerset TA6 6LQ
Telephone: (0278) 429089

ITALY
A.G.O.R.,
via Rancisvalle 70,
37136 Verona,
Telephone: 045 584 177

U.S.A.
A Chance to Grow,
5034 Oliver Avenue North,
Minneapolis,
Minnesota 55430,
Telephone: 612-521 2266

Sandler-Brown Consultants,
612 Fitzwatertown Road,
Willow Grove,
Pennsylvania 19090
Telephone: 215-657 5250